Case Studies in Legal Psychology

Eric Rassin

Case Studies in Legal Psychology

Psychological Perspectives on Criminal Evidence

Springer

Eric Rassin
Erasmus University Rotterdam
Rotterdam, The Netherlands

ISBN 978-3-031-44930-7 ISBN 978-3-031-44931-4 (eBook)
https://doi.org/10.1007/978-3-031-44931-4

This Springer imprint is published by the registered company Springer Nature Switzerland AG
The registered company address is: Gewerbestrasse 11, 6330 Cham, Switzerland

Paper in this product is recyclable.

Keywords

Psychological analysis of criminal evidence
Likelihood ratio approach to criminal evidence
Bayesian approach to criminal evidence
Crime stories and psychology
Legal psychology and evidence evaluation
Mistaken identifications
Eyewitness errors and false convictions
Interrogation tactics and false confessions
Miscarriages of justice

About the Book

In some criminal cases, it is a difficult challenge to find out what happened. Fact finders will rely on different approaches ranging from intuitive heuristics to scientific insights. With 11 real cases, this book illustrates how professional judges evaluate criminal evidence. Moreover, the legal psychological approach to the same evidence is discussed, as the author served as a psychological expert witness in these cases. Targeted pieces of evidence and related topics include:

- Eyewitness identification
- Eyewitness testimony
- Confession evidence
- Deception
- Memory flaws
- Legal decision making

It is a must-read for practitioners and graduate students in criminal law, forensic psychology, and legal psychology.

Contents

1 Introduction 1
1.1 Fact Finding in Criminal Procedure 1
1.2 Legal Decision-Making Theory 3
1.3 Flaws and Biases in Legal Decision Making 9
1.4 The Legal Psychologist as Expert Witness 19
References 26

2 The Armed Robbery and a Disputed Identification in a Mugshot Series 31
2.1 Varieties of Identification Procedures 32
2.2 Estimator Variables 33
2.3 How This Case Ended 34
References 36

3 The Armed Robbery and a Disputed Identification in a Line Up 37
3.1 Fifty Rules for a Proper Line Up Identification Procedure 37
3.2 The Identification Evidence in This Case 52
References 54

4 Popeye and an Obscure Mix of Identification Procedures 57
References 61

5 Delayed Allegation of Sexual Assault, Repression and Psychotherapy 63
5.1 Criteria-Based Content Analysis (CBCA) 63
5.2 Recovered Memories 68
5.3 Clinical Versus Legal Psychology 73
5.4 The Alternative Hypothesis 75
5.5 How the Case Ended 79
References 79

6 Dissociation as a State of Reduced Consciousness ... 83
6.1 Laypeople's Strange Beliefs About Psychological Treatment ... 83
6.2 The Verdict ... 87
References ... 87

7 The Tantra Therapist and the Threat of Collaborative Storytelling ... 89
References ... 92

8 Magic Mumfry and the Snowball Effect ... 93
8.1 The Effect of Rumours ... 93
References ... 96

9 A Shocked and Caring Community ... 97
9.1 The Information Session ... 97
9.2 Anatomically Detailed Drawings ... 100
9.3 How This Case Ended ... 104
References ... 104

10 The Amnestic Murderer ... 107
10.1 Memory Enhancement ... 108
10.2 Genuine or Simulated Amnesia ... 109
10.3 A Small Battle of Forensic Experts ... 118
References ... 121

11 The Breda Six ... 123
11.1 Interrogation ... 124
11.2 False Confession Experiments ... 128
11.3 Safeguards Against False Confessions ... 131
11.4 Negative Evidence ... 134
11.5 The End … or Is it? ... 134
References ... 135

12 Mister Big and a Disputed Confession ... 137
12.1 The Psychology of Confession ... 139
12.2 The Anatomy of Criminal Conviction ... 140
References ... 142

13 Conclusion ... 143
13.1 Case Studies as Starting Point of Analyses ... 143
13.2 Legal Psychology as a Forensic Expertise ... 144
13.3 Hypotheses-Driven Decision Making ... 150
References ... 153

Index ... 157

About the Author

Eric Rassin, Ph.D., M.L., is a professor of Psychology at Erasmus University Rotterdam, the Netherlands. His research focuses on legal decision making, biases, and credibility assessment. He has written over 100 scientific articles and 10 books. He serves as an expert witness in legal psychology regularly.

Chapter 1
Introduction

Over the past decades, I was asked to give psychological expert opinion in over 70 criminal cases. The topics on which opinion was solicited varied, but mainly revolved around the credibility of eyewitness statements, identification evidence, and confession evidence. In this book, I will discuss 11 of the cases in which I was involved. These cases were selected so as to serve as a starting point to discuss a psychological view on various pieces of criminal evidence. There is a rich tradition in psychological literature on various pieces of evidence, but the psychological view on evidence sometimes diverges from the legal view. Another selection criterion was that the cases were already published (at least in Dutch) online, so that all information can be found (in Dutch) on the internet (www.rechtspraak.nl). For every case, a case number is provided with which the case can be found. The fact that all cases are Dutch may result in typically Dutch legal peculiarities leaking though in the analyses. Nonetheless, the aim is to offer a universal approach to criminal evidence.

In this introductory chapter, legal fact finding and the position of the legal psychological expert witness are discussed. Next, 11 criminal cases will be discussed in separate chapters. Each chapter starts with a short factual description of the case. Next, a psychological perspective on the evidence will be given, intertwined with a discrete description of my contribution as an expert in the case. Finally, the court's verdict will be discussed to shed light on the anatomy of conviction.

1.1 Fact Finding in Criminal Procedure

What typically happens in a criminal investigation is that the police initially seek to identify a suspect. Once a primary suspect is in the picture, the police will seek to gather evidence against this suspect. It is not unusual to construe information both as preliminary information as well as incriminating evidence later on. For example,

E. Rassin, *Case Studies in Legal Psychology*,
https://doi.org/10.1007/978-3-031-44931-4_1

if the police have no suspect, and subject a witness to a photo series of previous suspects of similar crimes (a so-called mugshot series), and the witness identifies one of these photos, the pertinent suspect will then become the primary suspect in the present investigation. The same identification may later on, in court, be used as evidence against the suspect.

Once the police feel that they have gathered enough incriminating evidence against the suspect, they hand over the case to the public prosecution who will ultimately subpoena the suspect. Continental European Codes of Criminal Procedure are generally inquisitorial in nature. Consequently, the content of the casefile is for the bigger part determined by the public prosecution. However, the defence has some opportunity to include information (cf. exonerating evidence) in the file. Notwithstanding, generally, criminal casefiles contain mostly incriminating evidence. In fact, in Dutch, we only call information evidence if it is incriminating.

The casefile is subsequently sent to the court that will try the case. Prior to the trial, the judges will study the casefile. One of the main challenges during the trial is to establish facts, that is, it has to be proven that the suspect committed the crime of which he is suspected. If this is proven, it has to be decided what to do with the perpetrator. Which sanction is called for? He can be sentenced to imprisonment or receive another punishment. Instead or in addition, he can be sentenced to undergo treatment in a forensic clinic.

As to the first question, the judge (or jury) has all sorts of information at their disposal to be used as evidence, such as their own observations, witness statements including the casefile, other written documents and other files, statements given by the suspect, and advice given by expert witnesses. The use of information as evidence is bound by rules, and thus, so is legal fact finding. Consequently, criminal fact finding may not always result in discovering factual truth. One reason for this is that evidence may in some cases be inadmissible, because the police violated rules during their investigation. Moreover, the end goal of a criminal trial is to establish whether or not the suspect committed the crime at hand. This is not always the same as finding out what happened. For example, if the judge deems that it cannot be established that the suspect committed the crime, the judge is not obligated to find out who did. To that end, a new procedure has to be started.

At the end of the trial, the judge ultimately decides whether or not there is enough incriminating evidence to convict the suspect. There is consensus that conviction requires at least two, preferably independent, pieces of evidence. It is the judges' prerogative to select and evaluate these pieces of evidence. Imagine that there are two pieces of incriminating evidence in a casefile, but also eight pieces of exonerating evidence. Even in such situation, the judge can convict the suspect, referring to the two pieces of incriminating evidence, while ignoring the exonerating evidence. Hence, when finding facts, the judge is free to display some cherry-picking.

Note further that establishing that the suspect is the perpetrator does not require absolute proof, but merely sufficient evidence, so that perpetratorship can be assumed beyond reasonable doubt. In essence, it is simply assumed that when a(n unknown) threshold of evidence is reached, perpetratorship is proven.

Arguably, establishing perpetratorship, despite its legal context, is in fact not a legal expertise. It comes closer to a historical or scientific endeavour, rather than legal expertise. It can hence be argued that establishing perpetratorship requires historical and scientific, rather than legal methods. Obviously, judges are not typically trained in historical and scientific methodology. Thus, it can be argued that judges are from the onset ill-prepared to engage in fact finding. They may themselves disagree, if they fail to appreciate that law is fundamentally different from history or science. Strikingly, in Dutch (and other languages), it is impossible to distinguish science from arts and humanities. These academic disciplines are all referred to with the same overarching term. Haack (2003, p. 344) noted this and concluded: 'There are plenty of questions – historical, legal, logical, political, philosophical, commercial, culinary, etc., etc. – that simply fall outside the scope of the sciences (as that not-quite-translatable German word, Wissenschaft, is broader than science)'. In a similar vein, in Dutch, there is only one word for (scientific) research and (criminal) investigation. Further it is impossible to distinguish between evidence and proof. In sum, while standards for fact finding in criminal procedures are high, the standards are far from absolute.

1.2 Legal Decision-Making Theory

There is a handful of theories on how judges do and should find fact. First, there is theory borne out by regulation. For example, if the law dictates that one single piece of evidence does not suffice to convict a suspect, this implies that the decision to convict should rest on at least two pieces of evidence. Question then is whether every piece of evidence should support the whole indictment, or just one part of it. For example, if someone is murdered with a knife, and this knife is found at the suspect's home, this knife is one single piece of evidence. Legally, the dead body of the victim can now be construed as a second piece of evidence that supports the indictment in so far that a murder at least did take place (though not necessarily by the suspect).

Apart from "theory" that is in fact a consequence of legal doctrine and jurisprudence, there is a more psychologically oriented theory, known as the story model. Crucial to this theory is that information (whether a witness statement, a body, or a weapon) only becomes evidence if it fits in a story, that is, a convincing account of what happened (Pennington & Hastie, 1992). Further, according to the coherence-based reasoning viewpoint, independent pieces of evidence may cognitively interact if they both support the same story (Simon, 2004). Recent research suggests, for example, that if the decision maker is convinced of the suspect's guilt, (s)he will consider the evidence to be stronger, compared to when (s)he judges the strength of the evidence outside of the context of a specific case (see Greenspan & Scurich, 2016). The cognitive interaction between various pieces of evidence, or between evidence and story can have both beneficial effects, in that the evidence is given meaning by the context, and negative effects, in that the perceived strength of the evidence is artificially inflated due to the context information.

Wagenaar et al. (1993) proposed a normative theory from the prosecution's viewpoint. They argued that, for a case to be convincing, the incriminating story has to be supported with evidence at every crucial point. If a piece of evidence is disputable (e.g., an eyewitness identification that might be argued to be mistaken), this evidence needs additional evidence one level deeper (e.g., information about the identification procedure). This process of finding deeper level evidence should continue until the level of generally known facts that need no further elaboration is reached. In this way, the story of the indictment becomes anchored with evidence, and if needed, that evidence is anchored with additional evidence. Hence, this viewpoint is known as the theory of anchored narratives. It is illustrated in Fig. 1.1, in a fictitious case in which the victim was robbed by a stranger who threatened him with a knife, left at the crime scene.

A different account of legal decision making is the argumentative approach by Wigmore (1913). Arguably, the Wigmorian chart method is not so much a theory of legal decision making as a way to make complex evidence constellations clear in an elaborated chart. In a Wigmorian chart, that can spread over multiple pages, all known facts, evidence, and counterevidence are included. It is a flow chart in which the weight of information (e.g., known fact versus disputed evidence or assumption) can be manifested in different geometric figures (e.g., circles, squares, and triangles; Goodwin, 2000; Leclerc et al., 2022). A chart of our example of the armed robbery might look like Fig. 1.2.

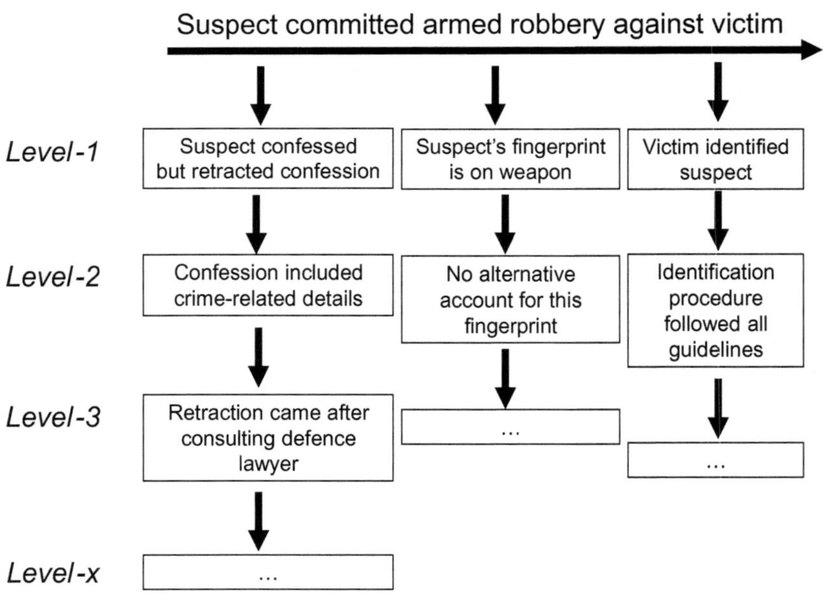

Fig. 1.1 Illustration of an anchored narrative. (Wagenaar et al., 1993)

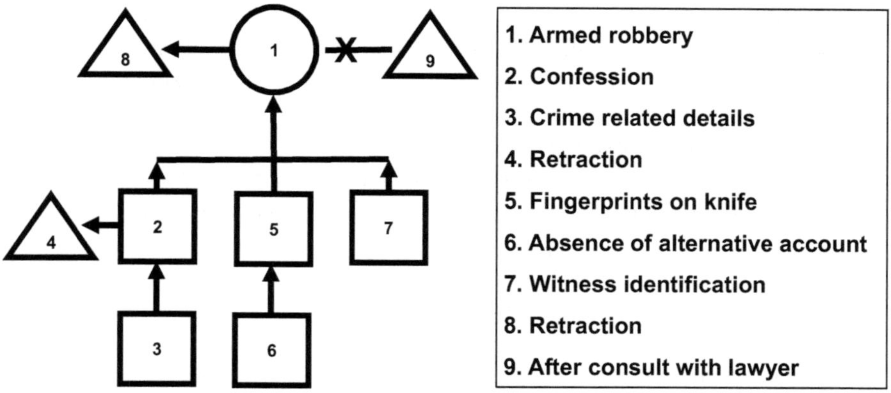

Fig. 1.2 Illustration of a (simplified) Wigmorian evidence chart

A final decision-making theory is the Bayesian approach to evidence. Crucial to this approach is that it is probabilistic. This approach goes back to reverent Thomas Bayes (1702–1761) of whom just one text has been retained in which he explains how one's belief in an undetermined phenomenon requires updating when encountering new information. This text was published by Bayes' friend Richard Price (1763) 2 years after Bayes had passed away.

In this text, Bayes explains how we can form and update believes about phenomena that we cannot observe directly. He used the analogue of throwing balls on a table. Imagine that we throw a ball on a table with our eyes closed. Imagine further that this ball (and others to follow) actually land(s) and remain(s) somewhere on the table without hitting anything else. We do not know where exactly ball 1 has landed. Now, a second ball is thrown on the table. If the first ball coincidentally has landed exactly in the middle of the table (this thought experiment is two-dimensional), there is 50% likelihood that the second ball lands to the left and 50% likelihood that it lands to the right side of ball 1. Imagine that the second ball lands on the left side of ball 1. Now, imagine that ball 3 also lands left of ball 1. We may now begin to suspect that ball 1 has landed somewhat to the right side of the table rather than exactly in the middle. The more balls keep up ending to the left of ball 1 (so we are told), the stronger our belief that ball 1 is on the right side of the table will become. With this analogue, Bayes explained how our belief in the unknown phenomenon (the location of ball 1) can be updated after each new piece of information. Hence, in this belief updating system, the initial belief is referred to as the prior odds, the informativeness of each new piece of information is expressed as a likelihood ratio, and the eventual, adapted belief is referred to as the posterior odds. Given that the prior odds is multiplied by each new likelihood ratio (LR), a general way to express the Bayesian analysis is as follows:

$$\text{Prior odds}^{*}\ \text{LR}\,1^{*}\ \text{LR}\,2^{*}\ \text{LR}\,3\ldots^{*}\ \text{LR}\,x = \text{posterior odd.}$$

Both odds and likelihood ratios are quotients. The odds are defined as the probability that the primary hypothesis is true, divided by the probability that the alternative hypothesis is true. The likelihood ratios are defined as the likelihood that the evidence occurs under the primary hypothesis divided by the likelihood that it occurs under the alternative hypothesis.

These definitions clarify the difference between odds and likelihood ratios. That is, odds reflect the relative belief in the veracity of the primary hypothesis, given the evidence:

$$(H_1 | E) / (H_2 | E),$$

whereas the likelihood ratio reflects the strength of the evidence, given the hypotheses:

$$(E | H_1) / (E | H_2).$$

In other words, the odds represent the relative *probability* that the primary hypothesis is true, whereas the likelihood ratio represents the relative *likelihood* that the evidence is found if the primary hypothesis is true.

A classic example of how a Bayesian analysis works is the taxi problem (e.g., Gigerenzer, 1991). In this problem, a hit-and-run accident has taken place at night. A witness, curiously called miss Prob, testifies that she saw a blue taxi cause the accident and flee the crime scene. Conveniently, in this town, there are only two kinds of taxis: Blue and yellow cabs. Of all cabs, 15% are blue and 85% are yellow. Thus, the base rate of blue taxis is small. Assume that it is known for certain that miss Prob can accurately distinguish blue from yellow cabs in 80% of the trials. How probable is it that the taxi involved in the car accident was blue? Various answers to the question are possible. For example, one might conclude that the taxi was blue (with 80% confidence) because the witness testified so. Alternatively, one might argue that the taxi was probably yellow (with 85% confidence) because most taxis simply are yellow. The first position solely relies on the evidence, ignoring the base rate (this stance is sometimes referred to as the prosecutor's fallacy; Thompson & Schumann, 1987), whereas the second solely relies on the base rate, ignoring the evidence (sometimes referred to as the defence attorney's fallacy). A Bayesian computation makes it possible to reconcile the base rate and the evidence given by miss Prob. In this computation, the prior odds of a blue taxi is (15% / 85% =) 0.176, and the likelihood ratio of miss Prob's testimony is (80% / 20% =) 4. The posterior odds is (0.176 * 4 =) 0.704. This odds can be transformed to a probability with the formula.

$$(\text{odds}^* 100) / (\text{odds} + 1),$$

which yields a probability of ((0.704 * 100) / (0.704 + 1) =) 41%.

Applied to our fictitious case of the armed robbery, the Bayesian approach requires that likelihoods are estimated for the three main pieces of evidence: The identification by the victim, the suspect's fingerprint on the knife found at the crime scene, and the confession. The primary hypothesis is that the suspect is indeed the perpetrator, the alternative hypothesis is that he is not. In essence, the analysis boils down to deliberating about the estimated likelihood that the robbery victim would recognise the robber (a true positive identification), and the likelihood that he would falsely identify the innocent suspect (false positive identification). For the fingerprint, a dactyloscopy may shed light on the match between the print found on the knife, and a print taken from our suspect, and compare this match likelihood with the likelihood that a random person's fingerprint would match the one found on the knife (the so-called random match probability; RMP). Finally, for the confession, the judge has to estimate what the likelihood is that a guilty suspect will confess, and what the likelihood is that an innocent suspect would confess. Imagine that, with some advice from various experts, the judge determines all these likelihoods to be as displayed in Table 1.1 (cf., Rassin & Israëls, 2014; Steblay et al., 2003).

These estimates yield likelihood ratios of (47 / 23 =) 2, (100 / 0.000001 =) 100,000,000, and (74 / 45 =) 1.6. The combined evidentiary power is hence (2 * 100,000,000 * 1,6 =) 320,000,000, which corresponds with a probability that the suspect is guilty of 99.9999999%.

This example illustrates strengths and problems of the Bayesian approach to criminal evidence. The main strength of the approach is that it forces the decision maker to explicitly consider two competing hypotheses (suspect is guilty versus suspect is innocent). This is far less or not at all so in the other approaches. Considering alternative hypotheses will raise the quality of the decision, in that it prevents the decision maker from being satisfied when the evidence simply fits well with the suspect's guilt (and thus provides evidence for that). The Bayesian approach raises the bar because the decision maker has to exclude that the evidence can also fit well in an alternative hypothesis. In some instances, this consideration of an alternative account will yield the insight that the evidence does indeed also fit well in an alternative account, and is not as strong as previously thought, even though it fits perfectly with the suspect being the perpetrator. A limitation of the Bayesian approach is that it relies on the assumption that all information can be caught in likelihoods. Further, a closer look at Table 1.1 reveals that the prior odds is missing. In the context of criminal procedure, there may be problems with prior odds. A practical objection is that it is sometimes difficult to estimate a prior. If the police in our example started their investigation with looking at 10 old robbery cases, then the prior odds for our suspect might be set at (1 out of 10 =) 0.11. However, in a

Table 1.1 Illustration of a Bayesian analysis

	Identification	Fingerprint	Confession
Likelihood if suspect is perpetrator	47%	100%	74%
Likelihood if suspect is innocent	23%	0.000001%	45%

considerable proportion of cases, it is quite difficult to determine at which point a person becomes the primary suspect, and thus, what the prior odds is. A legal theoretical objection against the prior odds is that priors higher than one are emotionally at odds with the presumption of innocence. A simple way to evade objections against the prior is to estimate it at 1, which makes it irrelevant to the computation of the posterior odds. Starting with a prior odds of 1 becomes less problematic with an increase in the number of strong pieces of evidence. Obviously, the more weight is brought to the equation by the likelihood ratios, the less influence the prior odds has. In the words of Fenton et al. (2013): ‘It is possible to avoid the delicate and controversial issue of assigning a subjective prior probability to the ultimate hypothesis if we instead are prepared to focus on the probabilistic value of the evidence’ (p. 68). Another limitation is that the multiplying of the components in the equation requires that all evidence is completely independent from each other. However, this may not always be so. Imagine that the police confront a denying suspect with the positive outcome of an eyewitness identification procedure, after which the suspect decides to confess (Hasel & Kassin, 2009). In that case, the confession is conditional upon the identification and does not fully contribute to the equation. Rather than multiplication, a Bayesian network would then be appropriate, which is very difficult to do without software (Fenton et al., 2016). A final challenge for the Bayesian approach is that while quantification makes things transparent, this also leads to new questions. For example, how high does the posterior odds have to be to establish perpetratorship beyond reasonable doubt? Is 99.9999999% enough? In an attempt to shed some light on this topic, Rassin (2017a) posed the question to a sample of 58 professional judges. On average, the participants reported to generally require 93.6% confidence to convict a suspect. However, a rephrased version of the question (i.e., “How large do you allow the percentage of miscarriages of justice to be?”) yielded a more conservative response. After reversed scoring, the mean turned out to be 98.7%. Some participants reported 100% certainty (i.e., 0% miscarriages of justice), but that is in Bayesian terms impossible.

In recent literature, there seems to be an osmosis between different theoretical approaches. In these hybrid models, the idea that the decision maker needs to explicitly compare the guilt-hypothesis with an alternative innocence-hypothesis is taken as starting point. But the models do not always require that each piece of evidence is allocated a likelihood ratio. Instead, in these scenario models, the idea is that the decision maker has to determine whether the evidence actually helps to discriminate between the guilt hypothesis (or scenario) and the innocence hypothesis or scenario (Bex et al., 2010; van Koppen & Mackor, 2020; Verhey et al., 2016). Meanwhile, in my admittedly limited experience, judges oftentimes limit themselves to simply establishing whether there is enough evidence (that is at least two independent pieces) that supports the hypothesis that the suspect is the perpetrator.

1.3 Flaws and Biases in Legal Decision Making

Regardless which approach is taken, there is always the risk of a false verdict. In particular, miscarriages of justice (i.e., the conviction of an innocent suspect) are considered detrimental. This is so, because, while it is unfortunate if a perpetrator remains unpunished, a false conviction does exactly that plus it causes an innocent person to get into serious problems. As Kassin (1997) argued in reference to Blackstone's ratio: 'In the context of a legal system founded on the ideal that it is better to acquit 10 guilty people than to convict 1 person who is innocent … the false positive error – although less frequent than the false negative – presents the more serious problem' (p. 224).

That said, there are multiple potential causes of miscarriages of justice. For one thing, the evidence can be corrupt. Saks and Koehler (2005) analysed the evidence in 86 verdicts that had later turned out to be miscarriages of justice (thanks to new DNA analyses), and found that various pieces of evidence were corrupt (see Fig. 1.3).

Besides corrupt evidence, flaws in the legal decision-making process can cause mistakes. For example, emotions may pose a threat to rational decision making in various ways, such as by shifting the decision in the direction of the emotion, by providing information that steers the decision, or by affecting the decision-making strategy. A study by Douglas et al. (1997) illustrates that effects of emotions may well occur in legal decision-making contexts. The authors found that mock jurors were affected by the inclusion of (no vs. black-and-white vs. full colour) crime scene pictures in the casefile, in that the explicitness of the evidence inflated conviction rates.

Notwithstanding the effect of emotions, a simple lack of knowledge of the evidentiary strength of information may affect legal decision making. Suspecting an antisuspect bias (police, prosecution, and maybe the court at least might think that there is a reasonable possibility that the suspect is guilty, if for no other reason,

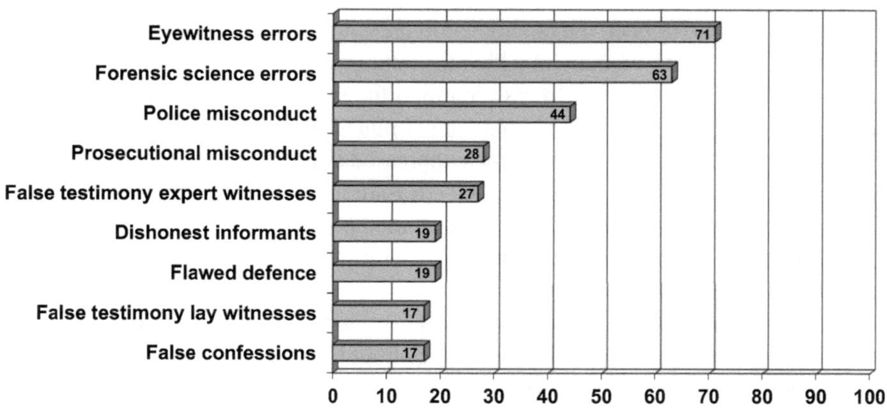

Fig. 1.3 Sources (%) of wrongful convictions. (Saks & Koehler, 2005)

because they all invested so much time and effort), incriminating evidence might be valued more than exonerating evidence. One example of a subtle skewed evaluation of evidence is that decision makers may tend to underestimate the exonerating power of negative evidence, that is, evidence that was searched for but not found. Imagine that the police expect to find incriminating evidence, ranging from drug residues in the blood of a rape victim, to fingerprints from the suspect on a murder weapon, but fail to find such evidence. Strictly theoretically, this failure to find the expected evidence may be construed as evidence against the hypothesis that the suspect is the perpetrator. However, there is some research suggesting that this negative evidence is sometimes simply discarded as irrelevant. One example of this phenomenon can be found in a study by Jenkins and Schuller (2007). They had 171 undergraduates read a case vignette about a drug facilitated sexual assault (DFSA). In this case, a man and woman met in the streets and recognised each other from high school. They went for a drink, and ended up having sex. The next day, the woman goes to the police and states that she was drugged and subsequently raped. The man denies this DFSA and testifies that he did not administer any drugs, and that all happened consensually. One third of the participants received additional information about a drug test taken by the woman. The outcome of this test was negative, that is, no residues of drugs were found. The remaining one third received, in addition to the negative drug test, a report about the oral questioning of the drugs expert. The expert testifies that the negative drug test does not prove that the woman had not been given drugs. The test was insensitive to 10% of known drugs. In the control condition (i.e., no drug test, no oral report), 14 out of 60 participants (i.e., 23%) chose to convict the suspect. Addition of the negative drug test suppressed conviction rate to 5 out of 57 (i.e., 9%). Strikingly, in the condition in which the added oral report gave room to mentally reduce the diagnosticity of the negative evidence, conviction rate inflated to 16 out of 54 (i.e., 30%). This finding suggests that negative evidence can have the logically expected effect, but is relatively easily discarded and even overcompensated. Unfortunately, in this experiment, the effect of negative evidence and its nuances was not compared to their positive counterparts (see also Thompson et al., 2017). The latter limitation was remedied in a study by Rassin (2013) who dubbed the phenomenon presence bias, in which 47 professional judges received a case vignette in which the outcome of an eyewitness identification test was either positive (the witness identified the suspect) or negative (the witness identified no-one). The positive outcome inflated conviction more (20 percent points) than that the negative outcome suppressed conviction (2 percent points). In addition, like Jenkins and Schuller (2007), Rassin found that participants tend to be better at explaining away negative outcomes than positive outcomes. Liebman et al. (2012) wrote a compelling argument, filled with real-life examples, for the appreciation of negative evidence.

The underappreciation of negative evidence and (other) exonerating evidence may not only result from limited knowledge about the strength of evidence, but also from flaws in logical reasoning. Take, for example, the premise 'A perpetrator will leave some kind of evidence at the crime scene'. This premise logically allows for the conclusion 'X commits a crime, and is apprehended because of evidence found at the crime scene' (modus ponens), but also for the conclusion 'No evidence against X is found, therefore he must be innocent' (modus tollens). By contrast, the conclusions 'X is innocent, and therefore no evidence against him will be found' (denial of the antecedent), and 'Evidence against X is found, therefore he is guilty' (affirmation by the consequent) are not (necessarily) logically valid. Note that the affirmation by the consequent fallacy is sometimes referred to as the transposed conditional, but also as the prosecutor's fallacy. It can be expected that people have difficulty with appreciating the logical validity of the modus ponens, and with understanding the invalidity of the transposed conditional/prosecutor's fallacy (Johnson-Laird, 1999). Indeed, Rassin (2018a) presented a premise, similar to the one discussed above, to a mixed sample of undergraduates ($n = 208$) and professional judges ($n = 40$). Next, the four conclusions were presented, and participants were asked to rate the logical validity of each on a scale from 0 (*completely invalid*) through 100 (*completely valid*). For the total sample ($N = 248$), the modus ponens was rated with a 76, while the modus tollens received an average of 41 (both ideally should be 100). The denial of the antecedent was rated with a 67, and the affirmation by the consequent with a 50 (both should be zero). Rassin also computed a composite variable: Modus ponens + modus tollens – denial of the antecedent – affirmation by the consequent. The score on this composite ranges from −200 (poor performance) through 200 (perfect performance). The mean score on the composite was 0.5, indicating that participants largely failed to appreciate the logical validity of the various conclusions. Notable, judges performed virtually the same as undergraduates.

In a second study, Rassin (2018a) had 71 undergraduates complete the same applied Wason (1968) card selection test (WCST) as in Study 1, and presented 41 of them with a case vignette based on an infamous Dutch miscarriage of justice. Participants indicated whether they would convict the suspect, based on the available evidence. Strikingly, the 22 participants who chose to convict the suspect scored worse on the composite variable (−6) than the 19 acquitting participants (9; $p < 0.05$). This suggests that logical thinking is associated with safer (i.e., suspect-friendlier) legal decision making. The remaining 30 participants read a fictitious case vignette in which there was strong evidence against the suspect (he and the victim had been locked in a house, his fingerprints were on the murder weapon, and he claimed to have been knocked out by a ghost). In this instance, convicting participants ($n = 26$) performed better on the WCST ($M = 8$) than did their four acquitting peers ($M = -31$; $p < 0.05$). Hence, superior performance on the WCST was not only associated with suspect-friendliness, but actually also with superior legal decision making.

Yet another reason for mistakes is that decision makers can be biased. A bias that has received some attention in the literature on legal decision making is the confirmation bias, defined as follows by Kassin: 'A warehouse of psychology research suggests that once people form an impression, they unwittingly seek, interpret, and create behavioural data that verify it' (2005, p. 219). As to the selective exposure to information that confirms one's prior hypothesis, Rassin et al. (2010) found in a sample of 79 undergraduates that decision makers who were convinced of the suspect's guilt were subsequently more interested in searching for additional incriminating evidence than those who were not convinced. More recently, similar findings were observed in a sample of 105 professional judges (Rassin, 2020).

Bias can be the result of exposure to context information, that is, information that is available to the decision maker but not probative for the determination of perpetratorship. This irrelevant information must be kept out of the deliberation. However, there is reason to argue that sometimes irrelevant information does affect the outcome of decision-making processes. A well-documented contextual effect on legal decision making is the order effect. That is, even though it should have no influence on the eventual conclusion, the order in which the decision maker processes the evidence does seem to affect the conviction. McKenzie et al. (2002) found an interesting order effect. In their second study, 120 undergraduates read a case vignette about a burglary in a warehouse. The suspect had a fairly weak defence, namely a befriended witness who gave him an alibi. The strength of the case for the prosecution differed. In the strong version, there was a positive eyewitness identification, the suspect had been convicted for multiple similar burglaries, and the method of entry was quite rare and identical to the one used by the suspect in previous instances. In the weak prosecution version, only the latter evidence was included. Participants rated their conviction of guilt on a scale from 0 (*certain of innocence*) through 20 (*certain of guilt*) on three occasions: At baseline, after the prosecution, and after the defence. Participants in the weak prosecution condition started around the midpoint of 10, shifted to 12 after the prosecution's case was presented, and dropped back to approximately 10 after the defence. In the strong prosecution condition, a different pattern emerged. Participants started at 10, rose to 13 after the prosecution, and rose further to almost 14 after the defence. Apparently, the strong case for the prosecution made the weak case for the defence appear so weak that it actually inflated, rather than slightly deflated, conviction. The authors argue that the evaluation of the exonerating evidence presented by the defence depends on the prior evaluation of the incriminating evidence presented by the prosecution. If the incriminating evidence is perceived as strong, the perceived strength of the exonerating evidence should meet a certain threshold to reduce conviction. If the exonerating evidence is weak, and does not meet this threshold, referred to as the minimum acceptable strength (MAS), a contrast effect will occur, and the weakness of the exonerating evidence may actually be perceived as incriminating, and will thus increase conviction.

Rassin (2017b) presented a case about a female suspect who might have murdered a psychiatrist to 53 professional judges. There were two versions, and in both, the evidence was the same (particularly, the suspect was found next to the victim, and her fingerprints were on the murder weapon). In one version, it was mentioned that the suspect had been diagnosed with severe psychopathy and antisocial personality disorder. Note that this diagnosis is relevant to the sentence, but it is not evidence of perpetratorship. Nonetheless, addition of the diagnosis inflated conviction rate from 46% to 79% ($p < 0.05$). This suggests that the order effect is most often a primacy effect, that is, prior information affects subsequent information. However, Kerstholt and Jackson (1998) argued that a recency effect might also occur, in that the most recently processed evidence is given disproportionally much weight. This may happen if the decision maker adjusts his belief by giving each new piece of information equal weight to his belief at that time, whereas in fact, the prior belief should weight heavier if it is based on multiple independent pieces of evidence.

Evidence order is not the only contextual effect that may hinder legal fact finding. Recently, Rassin (2020) combined a number of contextual effects in a sample of 105 professional judges. Participants read an adapted version of the casefile described by Rassin et al. (2010), and indicated whether they would convict the suspect. Unknown to the participants, there were two versions of the case, which did not differ in regard to the evidence, but in five nonprobative details, namely the severity of the injuries of the victim, the prior record of the suspect, the psychiatric diagnosis of the suspect, the order of the files (i.e., incriminating evidence first vs. exonerating evidence first), and the facial appearance of the suspect. Conviction rate was significantly higher in the suspect-unfriendly condition (i.e., 62%) than in the suspect-friendly condition (32%).

Various studies have yielded findings suggesting that context effects not only occur at the stage of conviction, but also during sentencing. Caruso et al. (2016) discovered that the use of slow motion recordings of the crime inflates perceived intent of the perpetrator. According to these authors, recordings are oftentimes played in slow motion (e.g., 2.25 times slower than regular speed) in court, in order to get a better look at the perpetrator. However, an unintended side effect is that the observer gets the impression that the perpetrator had more time to inhibit himself, and because he did not, perceived intent is inflated. Averaged over four experiments, 74% of regular speed viewers were convinced that the perpetrator carried out his criminal behaviour wilfully, compared to 82% of the viewers who saw the same recording but then in slow motion.

Sentencing might also be hindered by anchoring. Englich et al. (2005) presented a rape case to a mixed sample of 42 German professional judges and district's attorneys. In one version, the district's attorney demanded 34 months of imprisonment; in the other version, the demanded sentence was 12 months. The authors found that the sentence eventually chosen by participants was largely contingent on the demand of the district's attorney. That is, in the high demand condition, participants gave an average sentence of 27.6 months, and in the low demand condition, 19.3 months ($p < 0.005$). The content of the defence, including any alternative sentence proposal, was unrelated to the eventual verdict. Hence, the authors conclude that the sentence was solely and strongly anchored by the district's attorney's demand.

One year later, the same authors (Englich et al., 2006) elaborated further on the anchoring effect in the context of criminal sentencing. They presented a similar rape case as in their previous study (Englich et al., 2005) to 42 legal professionals. Before participants rendered their verdict, they were told to imagine that a journalist called them and asked whether the sentence would be lower or higher than 1 year. This question is irrelevant, because it stems from a journalist and does not dictate that the sentence should be lower or higher than 1 year. However, the question served to present a low anchor. Part of the participants received a version in which the journalist wondered whether the sentence would be lower of higher than 3 years (high anchor). Participants in the low anchor condition rendered a lower verdict (i.e., on average, 25 months), than did those in the high anchor condition (33 months; $p < 0.02$). In their final study, 52 legal professionals read a shoplifting casefile, and before rendering their verdict, they were told what the district's attorney's demand was. That is, the participant had to throw two dice, and the number of eyes thrown was to represent the number of months demanded by the district's attorney. This was done to make the participant fully aware that the demand was completely random, and not influenced by actual legal knowledge or guidelines. Unknown to participants, the dice were loaded so that half of the participants would throw three eyes (one plus two), whereas the other half always threw nine eyes (three plus six). Hence, participants were either exposed to a low (3) or high (9) anchor. Again, participants in the low anchor condition rendered a lower sentence (i.e., on average 5 months) than did those in the high anchor condition (i.e., 8 months; $p < 0.01$).

Wilson and Rule (2015) made a disturbing discovery when they analysed the facial appearance of capital crime convicts. They collected 742 photos of murder convicts. Half of them were sent to death row, the other half was sentenced to life imprisonment. Next, they asked 208 volunteers to rate the trustworthiness of the faces on a scale from 1 through 8. Strikingly, convicts on death row were perceived as less trustworthy (i.e., 2.76), compared to those who had received life imprisonment (i.e., 2.87; $p < 0.01$). While it is quite generally accepted that facial appearance is in fact not associated with actual trustworthiness, the authors ran a second study with 37 pictures of ex-convicts who turned out to have become the victim of a miscarriage of justice. These ex-convicts were found through the Innocence project website. Twenty had been sentenced to life imprisonment, and 17 to death sentence. The faces of these 37 innocent ex-convicts were rated for trustworthiness by 39 participants. Results of a logistic regression analysis confirmed that individuals with a less trustworthy appearance had been more likely to receive the death penalty. These findings constitute a clear example of a context effect, in that irrelevant information can indeed affect sentencing decisions.

Cho et al. (2017) sought to explore whether the slight sleep deprivation, caused by the forward spring shift to summertime, affects sentencing decisions on the Monday after the shift. They compared the sentences rendered on that sleepy Monday between 1992 and 2003 with comparison Mondays, and concluded that the average sentence on sleepy Monday was 5% longer.

A last example of contextual influences on legal decisions was provided by Danziger et al. (2011). They studied 1112 parole rulings on detention prolongation or termination, and found that the decisions were affected by the time of day at which they were ruled. That is, when the judges were fresh, at the start of the day, and after snack and lunch breaks, they were quite likely to terminate the detention, and thus, to rule in favour of the suspect (approximately 60% likelihood of termination). However, while working, the judges rapidly became increasingly likely to rule that detention should be maintained. Just before the break, the likelihood of termination dropped to nearly zero. Hence, these findings suggest that something as irrelevant as the time of day influences legal decision making. The authors explain their findings in terms of ego depletion. It should be noted that the judges in this study ruled 14 to 35 cases per day, sometimes leaving no more than 6 min per case to decide. It should also be noted that at the time of the ruling, the suspects were in detention. The authors argue that after some time, judges will suffer mental depletion, fatigue, and/or drop in blood sugar, and this will make it tempting to easily and safely maintain status quo. By contrast, after a break, the judges operate at full strength and have less problems with making relatively difficult decisions that diverge from the status quo (i.e., termination of detention).

One might argue that professional judges are better protected against flaws and biases than are lays, because of their experience and professional intuition. However, it must be acknowledged that some of the studies discussed in this paragraph leaned on samples of professional judges and did produce evidence of bias. Further, if decisions made by professional judges are fundamentally different from those made by lay juries, this should be traceable in scientific studies. Findings in a classic study by Kalven and Zeisel (1966) do not support the notion that professional judges have any kind of good intuition. They asked 3576 professional criminal trial judges for their opinion on the guilt of the suspect, in jury trials. In 78% of the cases, the judge would have ruled the same as had done the jury. Of the 22% of rulings that differed between judge and jury, 19% was caused by the judge believing that the suspect was guilty whereas the jury had chosen to acquit him. In 3%, the pattern was reversed: In these instances, the jury had ruled a guilty verdict whereas the judge would have chosen to acquit the suspect. It should be noted that the judge might sometimes have conformed to the ruling of the jury. Notwithstanding, Kalven and Zeisel (1966) argue: 'Presumably the judge, in general, would find it more comfortable to report agreement. If, therefore, he nevertheless reports disagreement, it seems only reasonable to accept this statement' (p. 51). Hence, the authors do not seem surprised that the agreement between judge and jury (i.e., 78%) was considerable, while in fact this agreement supports the idea that judges have no special intuition that makes them decide differently from lays. Moreover, in the majority of cases in which there was disagreement (i.e., 19% vs. 3%), the jury was more suspect-friendly than was the judge, while suspect-friendliness is arguably good in the light of the presumption of innocence. To evade the potential problem of judges conforming to jury rulings, the authors should have asked judges' opinion before the juries gave their ruling. However, they understandably argue: 'It would have been extravagant to arrange for a staff of interviewers throughout the United States to personally interview a judge each time he finished a jury trial' (p. 46, 47). Finally, Kalvin and Zeisel obtained similar results (i.e., 78% agreement) in 'a comparable sample of some four thousand civil jury cases' (p. 63). In short, these findings leave little room to argue that professional judges have developed a special kind of fruitful intuition enabling them to reach exclusive, special conclusions while rendering verdicts.

More recently, Rassin (2016) sought to explore whether good intuition fuels legal decision making, and/or bad intuition is detrimental to legal decision making. In a first study, 103 undergraduates completed four measures of intuition and rationality, and subsequently read a case vignette about a murder. They had to indicate whether they would convict the suspect. The intuition/rationality measures were the previously discussed RAT (Bowers et al., 1990), which measures good intuition, the

CRT (Frederick, 2005) measuring bad intuition, and the self-reported REI (Pacini & Epstein, 1999). The fourth measure was the critical thinking questionnaire (CTQ) adopted from Becker et al. (2007). The CTQ consists of 30 items measuring various aspects of critical thinking, namely, inference, interpretation, deduction, evaluation of arguments, and recognition of assumptions. One example is the following assignment. 'Imagine that disorder X occurs in one in every 1,000 people. Imagine also there is a test to diagnose the disorder that always gives a positive result when a person has the disorder. Finally, imagine that the test has a false positive rate of 5 percent. This means that the test wrongly indicates that the disorder is present in 5 percent of the cases where the person does not have the disorder. Imagine that we choose a person randomly, administer the test, and that it yields a positive result (indicates that the person has the disorder). What is the probability that the individual actually has the disorder, assuming that we know nothing else about the individual's psychological or medical history? A) <10%, B) 10–30%, C) 30–50%, D) 50–70%, E) 70–90%, F) >90%'. In this case, the correct answer is A. For every correct answer, 1 point is scored. Hence, the total score on the CTQ ranges from 0 through 30, with higher scores indicating higher levels of rational thinking. Findings indicated that participants who chose to convict the suspect scored lower on the CRT and on the CTQ. In a second study, a mixed sample of undergraduates, academic staff, and professional judges ($N = 94$) were brought in a rational or intuitive state by exposure to distinct pictures of, for example, Rodin's Le penseur (the thinker) versus Myron's Discus thrower. Next, they read a case vignette about a rape, and decided on the suspect's guilt. Participants brought in a rational state were less likely to convict the suspect (i.e., conviction rate was 34.1%) than those in which an intuitive state was induced (60%; $p < 0.03$). In the third experiment, 47 professional judges read a robbery case vignette. Half of them were instructed that when evaluating the evidence, they should realise that each piece of evidence has a true and false positive likelihood. This instruction was meant to induce a rational attitude. The other half were instructed to rely on their professional intuition. Again, participants in the rational condition displayed a lower conviction rate (43.5%) than those in the intuitive condition (75%; $p < 0.01$). In all, while intuition is difficult to study scientifically, the present findings suggest that (bad) intuition (e.g., low scores on the CRT and CTQ) is associated with increased conviction, while there is no reason to argue that good intuition (RAT, manipulated professional intuition) is associated with decreased conviction.

In conclusion, there is reason to argue that flaws and biases lure in the context of legal decision making. Interestingly, some authors argue that particularly the Bayesian approach to evidence may help reduce threats to valid legal decisions (e.g., Heuer, 1999; Liebman et al., 2012). This is so because the explicit consideration of an alternative hypothesis should reduce tunnel vision. Further, this approach makes the exonerating value of information explicit, because such information will have a likelihood ratio that is smaller than one, and is thus more likely under the innocence than under the guilt hypothesis.

It remains to be seen to what extent Bayesian and looser hybrid models actually raise the quality of judges' decision making, and offer protection against bias. In general terms, that requires that the decision maker is aware of the bias and its magnitude and direction, and is motivated to correct the bias, and able to adjust his strategy. Feigenson and Park add: 'Legal decision makers may fail to satisfy any or all of these criteria' (2006, p. 156). For starters, it may be difficult to appreciate the importance of considering alternative hypotheses. Second, it may be difficult to conjure up credible alternative hypotheses. Crucially, the primary and the alternative hypotheses must be mutually exclusive: They cannot both be simultaneously true. Hence, increase of confidence in one hypothesis must by definition detract confidence in the other (McKenzie, 1997, 1998, 1999). Kerstholt and Eikelboom (2007) presented 38 professional crime analysists with case vignettes, for example about a young woman from a strict religious background who went missing. Based on the evidence in the case, it was most likely that she had run away from home to go live with her Tunisian friend abroad. Participants were asked to generate as many hypotheses as possible about what might have happened. They also indicated which of these self-generated hypotheses they thought was the best, and worth most pursuing. Before doing this, half of the analysists were informed what the hypothesis of the investigating team was, namely that the woman had been murdered by her father who could not accept that she had a Tunisian friend. Of the naïve participants, 46% mentioned the father hypothesis, and 11% of them indicated that this particular hypothesis was the most likely. Of the group who had been informed about the father hypothesis, 94% mentioned it, and 39% believed that this was the most likely one. These findings suggest that knowing the primary hypothesis makes it difficult to generate alternatives.

Third, even if decision makers are presented with alternative hypotheses, they sometimes fail to see their importance. Mynatt et al. (1993) presented 107 undergraduates with a problem in which there were two alternatives and two sources of information. For example: 'Your sister has a car she bought a couple of years ago. It's either a car X or a car Y, but you can't remember which. You do remember that her car does over 25 miles per gallon and has not had any major mechanical problems in the two years she's owned it. You have the following piece of information: 1) 65% of car Xs do over 25 miles per gallon. Three additional pieces of information are also available: 2) The percentage of car Ys that do over 25 miles per gallon, 3) The percentage of car Xs that have had no major mechanical problems for the first two years of ownership, 4) The percentage of car Ys that have had no major mechanical problems for the first two years of ownership. Assuming you could find out only one of these three pieces of information (2, 3, or 4), which would you want in order to help you decide what car your sister owns?' In this situation, the most diagnostic information is number 2, because that will enable one to compare the percentages of cars that run over 25 miles per gallon. However, only 28% of the participants chose this information. Most participants (i.e., 51%) opted for number 3, that is, additional evidence for the first alternative. In their second study, the authors presented 101 undergraduates with versions of the problems in which the percentages (e.g., 65%) were replaced by percentages lower than 50% (i.e., 35%). In this instance, the percentage of participants who selected number 2 rose to 47%. This shift is striking because when considering alternative hypotheses, a likelihood of one (whether high, 65%, or low, 35%) is uninformative without the corresponding likelihood of the alternative.

Fourth and finally, if a decision maker is straight out confronted with an alternative hypothesis, he may still not know what to do with it. In a study by Ask and Granhag (2005), 50 police officers read a story about a murdered psychiatrist. The primary suspect, Eva, was found next to the victim, and the murder weapon, a knife, had her fingerprints on it. In the motive version, it was mentioned that Eva had expressed suspicion about her man who was a client of the psychiatrist, having an affair with the victim. In the alternative suspect condition, participants were instead informed that the victim had received threatening phone calls from an unknown man, probably an ex-client, who threatened to kill her. Participants indicated to what extent they were convinced that Eva was guilty on a scale from 0 through 9. While at first sight participants in the alterative suspect condition were less convinced ($M = 5.7$) than those in the motive condition ($M = 6.4$), this difference was nonsignificant ($p = 0.16$). Interestingly, in a replication in a sample of 68 undergraduates, the average conviction in the alternative suspect condition ($M = 5.0$) was significantly lower than that in the motive condition ($M = 6.3$; $p < 0.001$). In a replication in another mixed sample of 58 police officers, 16 district's attorneys, and 44 judges, Rassin (2010) found no difference in conviction rate between the motive condition (i.e., 13%) and the alternative suspect condition (12%; $p = 0.46$). Again, the group difference in a student sample ($N = 178$) did reach significance ($p < 0.05$) with 38% conviction rate in the motive condition, and 21% in the alternative suspect condition. O'Brien (2009) gave a case description about a shooting to 108 undergraduate students. In this story, there were multiple potential suspects, but one, Bill Briggs, was incriminated most by circumstantial evidence. After reading the case, some participants were asked to register their initial impression about who the perpetrator was. Then, they could select additional lines of investigation from a list of 25, some of which were incriminating for Briggs, whereas others were aimed at findings evidence against another suspect. Findings indicated that participants who were initially under the impression that Briggs was guilty selected more ($M = 1.65$) guilt confirming investigations than did those who had not expressed their initial suspicion ($M = 1.31$; $p < 0.05$). In a second study ($N = 109$ undergraduates), part of the participants again expressed their initial suspicion, but some of them also had to list three other potential suspects. Others had to list, besides their initial suspicion, reasons why they might be mistaken and why the primary suspect could be innocent. Hence, there were four conditions. As to the number of subsequently selected investigations aimed at gathering more evidence against Briggs, participants in the control condition selected on average 1, those in the initial hypothesis condition 1.48, those who had additionally listed three alternative suspects 1.54, and those who had thought of reasons why the suspect might be innocent 1.07. These data suggest that considering alternative suspects did not suppress confirmation proneness, whereas thinking of counterarguments for one's hypothesis did. Arguably, it is understandable that decision makers will become more eager to find evidence against the primary suspect after having considered three alternative suspects. Meanwhile, considering counterarguments can be construed as a form of alternative hypotheses thinking. It should be noted that in some legal systems, it is made difficult if not impossible for the defence to argue that there are alternative suspects (Findley & Scott, 2006; Liebman et al., 2012).

Given the apparent limited effect of (hybrid) alternative hypotheses thinking, Rassin (2018b) sought to explore whether it helps to literally type out the two competing hypotheses and to score the fit of each piece of evidence within both hypotheses, thus more closely resembling a Bayesian approach. Undergraduates ($N = 277$) read a version of Ask and Granhag's (2005) murder story about Eva and the killed psychiatrist. One third of the participants read the motive version, one third read a version in which both Eva's motive and the alternative male suspects were presented, and one third read the latter version, and was subsequently instructed to rate 20 pieces of information on their fit in the primary and in the alternative hypothesis, on a scale from 0 through 10. Finally, participants decided whether Eva should be convicted. In the motive condition, conviction rate was 36%. In the mixed motive and alternative suspect condition, conviction rate was suppressed to 22%, but this decrease was not statistically significant. In the pen-and-paper tool condition, conviction rate was significantly suppressed to 5% ($p < 0.001$). In a second study, findings were replicated employing a sample of 45 criminal justice professionals, and a within-subject design. Participants read the mixed motive and alternative suspect version of the case description, and subsequently indicated whether the suspect should be convicted. Next, they completed the pen-and-paper task also used in Study 1. Finally, they decided again whether they would convict the suspect. In this instance, conviction rate at T 1 was 22%, and (after assigning a fit between 0 and 10 under both hypotheses for each of 20 pieces of evidence) at T 2, significantly ($p < 0.04$) suppressed to 7%.

1.4 The Legal Psychologist as Expert Witness

Psychologists can be asked for advice in various stages of a criminal investigation. If the police ask for assistance with identifying a suspect or with finding evidence against the suspect, the psychologist will serve as an investigative psychologist. If the judge, defence, or prosecution asks for an opinion on the strength of evidence in the context of fact finding, this opinion can be called a legal psychological advice. Finally, psychologists who give opinion about the criminal responsibility of the suspect or other mental health related topics can be referred to as forensic psychologists. Legal psychologists give advice on the strength of nontechnical pieces of evidence including witness statements, eyewitness identification evidence, and confessions. They have various strategies at their disposal. One strategy is to study what can be called symptomatic expressions of the to-be-evaluated piece of evidence. For example, if the validity of a child-witness statement is disputed, the legal psychologist might use Criteria Based Content Analysis (CBCA; Steller & Köhnken, 1989) to see to what extent the statement includes cues associated with validity such as detailedness and logical consistency. Likewise, the expert witness might give attention to the self-reported confidence of a witness who identified the suspect in an identification procedure (Wells et al., 2020). As another example, the validity of a confession might be estimated by counting the number of crime-related details in it. A second strategy is to have the individual who produced the evidence take psychological tests. For example, in case of disputed confession evidence, the confessing suspect might be subjected to Gudjonsson's Suggestibility Scale (GSS: Gudjonsson, 1984). A high score on suggestibility may contribute to the argument that the suspect falsely confessed, because of his vulnerability to suggestion, allegedly made during the police interrogation. A third strategy is to identify crucial incidents in the development that have resulted in the evidence to occur. For example, legal psychologists may discuss the effects of delay and post hoc influences on memory. To this end, the history of the case as evident from the casefile, is of importance.

As with legal decision making, expert opinion has been shown to be susceptible to bias. At first sight, this might seem strange, because expertise and bias do not seem to go together, but the literature says different. Indeed, various biases have been documented in the work of experts from all sorts of domains, including DNA analysis, fingerprint analysis (dactyloscopy), bone analysis (anthropology), bite marks (odontology), bloodstain analysis, handwriting and voice analysis, toolmark and bullet analysis (ballistics), and pathology (see for a review, Cooper & Meterko, 2019). Kassin et al. even speak of a forensic confirmation bias defined as 'the class of effects through which an individual's preexisting beliefs, expectations, motives, and situational context influence the collection, perception, and interpretation of evidence during the course of a criminal case' (2013, p. 45). A spectacular example was provided by Dror et al. (2005) who asked 27 undergraduates to perform match decisions on 96 pairs of fingerprints. Part of the pairs were obvious matches or nonmatches whereas others were ambiguous (see Fig. 1.4 for examples). Some pairs were presented blindly, that is, without any context information. Others were accompanied by nonemotional information (e.g., a picture of a neutral part of the crime scene); a third group of pairs was presented together with emotional context information (e.g., a bloody picture of the victim), and the last class of pairs was accompanied by emotional context and subliminal messages such as 'same' or 'guilty'. Whereas the decisions regarding the unambiguous pairs were not affected by context, those regarding the ambiguous pairs were indeed influenced: Matches were concluded in 46% of the pairs without context, in 49% of the nonemotional

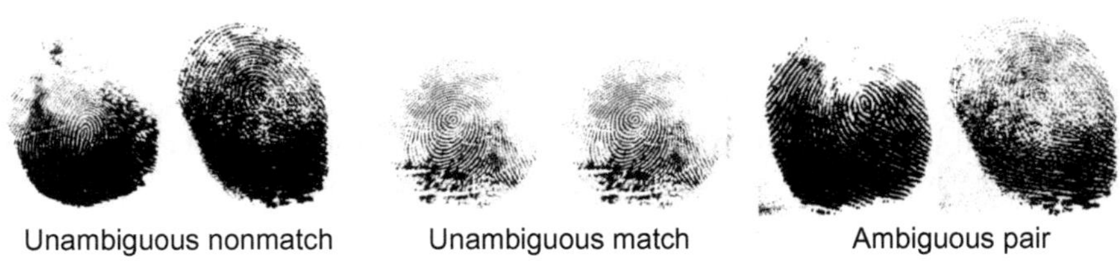

Fig. 1.4 Fingerprint examples after Dror et al. (2005)

context pairs, in 58% of the emotional context pairs, and in 66% of the emotional context plus subliminal messages pairs ($p < 0.001$). Hence, these findings suggest that context information can indeed increase perceived matches in fingerprint analyses.

The same research group also found evidence to suggest that factual matches can be made to be missed, by providing context information. In this particular study, a small group of professional fingerprint experts were included (Dror et al., 2006). It is somewhat ironic that fingerprint analyses are vulnerable to context effects and bias, because fingerprints are considered to be extremely unique and thus construe very strong evidence of identity. Here, there is a mismatch between practical utility and scientific rigour. On the one hand, we "know" that fingerprints are unique and at the same time consistent. Therefore, they are used for identification purposes in criminal proceedings, but also as digital keys. On the other hand, the whole idea of the uniqueness of fingerprints goes back to a classic study by Francis Galton (1892) and leans on nothing more than a case series in a few dozens of participants. Lilienfeld and Landfield (2008) even go as far as to attribute characteristics of pseudoscience to dactyloscopy. Then again, even though the hypotheses that the sun always comes up again, and that human life is fleeting are impossible to test experimentally and are actually based on a long series of cases, and are thus scientifically weak, it would be almost ridiculous to refute them.

Richards et al. (2015) introduced the diagnosis momentum bias, which refers to the situation in which experts (e.g., psychologists) tend to stick to a psychiatric diagnosis, and revolve their subsequent work around that diagnosis, without realising that diagnoses are sometimes incorrect, and even if they are correct, test scores may fluctuate naturally, and therefore one test result is not sacred and should not steer all the subsequent analyses. Another potential pitfall for experts is the outcome bias (Baron & Hershey, 1988). Imagine an oncologist who is charged for missing a cancer node during a routine screening. If the court appoints an expert (i.e., a colleague oncologist) to advise on the gravity of missing the tumour, this expert knows that the to-be-evaluated scan contains an irregularity. This prior knowledge may be difficult to ignore when evaluating the miss of the oncologist. Hence, knowing the unfortunate outcome (i.e., the development of a tumour that might have been prevented if it had been detected during the screening) will make the expert more readily conclude that the miss construes a breach of professional standards. Indeed, Hofvind et al. (2005) found that 35.9% of initially missed cancers were in hindsight classified by informed experts as such, while only 19.9% were classified as such by experts who were blind for the history of the scans at the time they evaluated them (i.e., they were simply asked to inspect the scans for suspicious nodes).

In addition, experts may be susceptible to what has been referred to as allegiance bias (Murrie et al., 2013) or financial bias (Richards et al., 2015). That is, the tendency to write a report that is beneficial to the commissioning party. The threat of allegiance bias seems more real in civil than in criminal cases, and more in adversarial (where each party can bring their own expert) than in inquisitorial systems (where experts are oftentimes directly hired by the court), but it lures in every situation. Note that in many fields of expertise, there is scientific discussion, and thus, an expert can choose to interpret information in one way or another. There is room for differential focus and emphasis. Richards et al. (2015) add that retaining parties might put some pressure on the expert to produce a favourable report. Such pressure might be hard to detect when it takes the form of a question to rephrase a certain part of the report allegedly to make it clearer to non-expert lawyers.

Interestingly, while there is ample evidence in the literature of bias in expert decisions, some experts themselves disagree that they are at risk of making biased decisions. Kukucka et al. (2017) asked a mixed sample of 403 professional experts from the field of DNA, fingerprint, handwriting, toxicology, and ballistics whether they believed that bias is a cause for concern in forensic science as a whole. This question was answered affirmatively by 71% of the participants. When asked whether bias is a cause for concern in their own specific domain, 52% replied confirmatively. But when asked whether their own judgments are influenced by bias, only 26% confirmed the question. Hence, people seem to have a bias blind spot. Meanwhile there is no reason to argue that particularly psychologists are less susceptible to bias than others.

In some forensic science domains, remedies have been sought to protect practitioners against bias. One main strategy is that the expert needs to be shielded from as much contextual information as possible. This can be achieved by blind testing, that is, the expert should only receive materials that are required to complete his analysis. All other information is redundant and should be kept from him to prevent contextual influences (Kassin et al., 2013). Experts that work in teams may want to have one expert do the intake with the commissioning party, while a colleague performs the actual analysis.

Another safeguard is that experts should employ multiple comparison methods (Cooper & Meterko, 2019) also referred to as evidence line ups (Kassin et al., 2013). That is, when detecting a match in handwriting between a threatening letter and a text written by the suspect, for example, the expert should not solely compare these two texts, but should include foils written by third parties. Ironically, this notion is relatively new in the hard beta forensic sciences, but was already proposed in legal psychology decades ago by Wagenaar (1989) who, admittedly, could lean on even older work (van Asch van Wijck, 1937).

The most drastic procedural change in the work of expert witnesses aimed at protection against bias is that they report their findings in a likelihood ratio format. By now, many forensic scientists in, for example, Europe and Australia have adopted this approach (Thompson, 2018; Thompson et al., 2018). Several professional associations and standard-setting bodies advise or even dictate the inclusion of likelihood ratios in expert reports (Association of Forensic Science Providers [AFSP], 2009; European Network of Forensic Science Institutes [ENFSI], 2016). Advocates of likelihood ratios see various advantages of the approach. For example, the AFSP (2009) mentions as underlying guiding principles: Balance (i.e., at least two competing hypotheses need to be included in the analysis), logic (likelihood ratios force the expert to reason prospectively), robustness (likelihood ratios ideally follow from scientific research, and they are fixed), and transparency (it is clear on what the expert's opinion is based). Implied in these guiding principles is a protection against various biases that threaten the validity of the expert opinion. For example, by comparing the likelihood of the to-be-evaluated piece of evidence within two competing hypotheses, the risk of falling prey to confirmation bias or tunnel vision is suppressed. Further, given that likelihoods are based on solid research, the risk of allegiance bias is reduced (numbers are fixed and cannot be bent).

There are various reasons to argue that legal psychologists should also adhere to the advice to report likelihoods. First, the mentioned advantages will apply to psychological expert opinion (Rassin et al., 2022). Second, the AFSP dictated in 2009 that 'across all scientific disciplines' (p. 161), 'the opinion or conclusion should express the degree of support for one proposition or the other depending upon the value of the likelihood ratio' (p. 163) and thus depends on 'the estimation of a likelihood ratio' (p. 161). Arguably, psychology is a science. Third, long before the paradigm shift that introduced the likelihood ratio in the forensic sciences (Saks & Koehler, 2005), it was a legal psychologist, no less, who advocated the inclusion of likelihood ratios in psychological expert opinion (Wagenaar, 1988). He forwarded an additional advantage of using likelihood ratios. To appreciate his argument, imagine an expert who uses the CBCA, 'probably the most widely used veracity assessment technique in the world' (Oberlader et al., 2016, p. 441), to estimate the validity of a witness statement. Beware that CBCA is an entirely one-dimensional checklist, with anchor points being *testimony is not credible* and *testimony is credible*. With this instrument, the expert simply checks to what extent the provided statement meets specific criteria (such as detailedness and spontaneousness), and then advises on its credibility. Any alternative hypothesis (e.g., that the witness is mistaken, or lying) is merely addressed implicitly. Thus, if the expert concludes that the statement is credible, this implies that it is likely to be true, and thus unlikely to be false. In doing so, the CBCA seduces the expert to give an opinion about the probability that the primary hypothesis is true, which is actually the prerogative of the judge or jury. Wagenaar (1988) warned that if social scientists do not employ a likelihood ratio format, there is a 'danger that social scientists will misrepresent the reliability of their knowledge and make biased statements' (p. 499). By including likelihood ratios, the different roles of expert and judge become clearly visible. The expert can say something about the likelihood of obtaining the evidence under two competing hypotheses (E | H). The judge has to determine which of the two hypotheses is most likely the correct one considering all the evidence (H | E).

Unfortunately, likelihood ratios have their limitations. First, the concept seems difficult to understand. De Keijser and Elffers (2012) tested the understanding of likelihood ratios in a mixed sample of 285 professionals (118 judges, 69 defence lawyers, and 98 forensic experts). They presented participants with two case vignettes about robberies in both of which a forensic analysis in likelihood ratio format was included. They then asked participants how well they understood these reports on a scale from 1 through 7. Besides this self-reported understanding, they sought to test actual comprehension with eight statements of which the participants had to decide whether they followed from the report or not. Some of the statements were indeed logically valid (e.g., 'The findings of this research make up strong evidence against the suspect'); others did not follow from the report (e.g., 'It is more likely that the suspect is guilty than innocent'). With these eight statements, participants could achieve a score between zero (poor understanding) and eight (proper understanding). The unweighted average self-reported and actual comprehension in the whole sample were 5.57 and 4.58, respectively. Hence, while self-reported understanding was satisfactory, proper understanding was not. More recently, Rassin et al. (2022) let the same instruments loose on a sample of 79 professional judges and obtained more promising results, that is, 6.35 on self-reported understanding (anchors 0 through 10) and 5.45 on proper understanding (anchors 0–8).

As to the difficulty of the concept of likelihood ratios, Martire et al. (2013) discovered an obscure phenomenon, namely that the verbal expression for small likelihood ratios (1–10), weak support, may have a reverse effect. The authors presented a case vignette about a theft to 75 undergraduates. Among the evidence was an expert analysis of a footprint left by the thief. In the different versions of the case vignette, the likelihood ratio for this footprint was either 4.5, 450, or 495,000. Half of the participants were given the corresponding verbal description instead of the numeric expression (i.e., weak support, moderately strong support, or very strong support, respectively). Participants were asked to indicate to what extent they believed that the suspect was guilty, in the format of an odds ('Based on the available evidence I believe that it is … times more likely that the accused is guilty than not guilty') twice; once before and once after reading the expert witness report. In this way, the authors could test the effect of the expert report on conviction. As can be expected, in most conditions, participants were more convinced of the suspect's guilt after reading the report, compared to before. The increase in conviction was similar in participants who received the numeric or the verbal description. There was one exception: Participant who read that the likelihood ratio was 4.5 displayed an increase of 1.35, whereas those who read that the likelihood ratio provided weak support displayed a decrease in conviction (−1.39). Hence, the phrase 'weak support' was erroneously interpreted as evidence against the primary hypothesis. Martire et al. (2013) dubbed this the weak evidence effect.

A second limitation of likelihood ratios is that they require that all information be reduced to likelihoods. For technical analyses (e.g., fingerprints and DNA), this is generally accepted, but for complex phenomena such as human behaviour, this reduction meets much resistance. Note that it is relatively new (i.e., since decades) that people have become accustomed to the idea that findings in psychological research can by deduction be used to make estimates in individual cases (Walker & Monahan, 1987).

A third challenge for the use of likelihood ratios in legal psychology is that the multicausality of behaviour causes the true positive likelihoods to be relatively modest, the false positive likelihoods to be relatively high, and consequently, the likelihood ratios to be relatively low. Note that in technical analyses at the source or identity level, likelihood ratios can run in the billions. To illustrate, Table 1.2. presents likelihood ratio ranges and their verbal descriptions, common in technical domains. Admittedly, in evidence subjected for analysis by legal psychologists, the likelihood ratios rarely exceed 100. Interestingly, technical analyses at the activity level suffer from that same problem. Kokshoorn et al. (2017) argue: 'More often

Table 1.2 Likelihood ratio ranges (AFSP, 2009)

Verbal description	Likelihood ratio
Weak support	1–10
Moderate support	10–100
Moderately strong support	100–1000
Strong support	1000–10,000
Very strong support	10,000–1000,000
Extremely strong support	1000,000<

Table 1.3 Likelihood ratio ranges (Rassin et al., 2022)

Verbal description	Likelihood ratio
Weak/anecdotal support	2–3
Positive/substantial support	3–10
Positive/strong support	10–30
Strong/very strong support	30–100
Very strong/decisive support	100<

than not, the source of DNA traces found at the crime scene is not disputed, but the activity or timing of events that resulted in their transfer is' (p. 115). For example, in most cases, in the 'old days', a strong DNA likelihood would construe evidence that the suspect was the perpetrator. However, by now, in general, defence attorneys have found their way to alternative hypotheses that allow for such a DNA likelihood. For example, a defence attorney may argue that DNA of his client may well have been found at the crime scene (a robbed shop), because the client had visited the shop merely as a customer, prior to the robbery. With this alternative account, the DNA does not prove that the suspect is the perpetrator. Compared to identity/source analyses, analyses at the activity level are much more complex, because they are determined by many more factors such as the possible retention of the trace under various external circumstances (e.g., was the shop cleaned between the alleged visit by the suspect and the robbery? If so with which detergent?). Likelihood ratios at the activity level are much lower than those at the source level. As such, the research needed to estimate activity level likelihoods, and the resulting ratios come closer to what legal psychologists are used to.

Considering that likelihood ratios in non-technical analysis (and in technical analyses at the activity level) are relatively modest, we recently proposed alternative likelihood ratio ranges and verbal descriptions (Rassin et al., 2022). These are presented in Table 1.3.

Finally, a few notes on the content and form of legal psychological expert witness reports must be made. Recently, Vredeveldt et al. (2022) presented the following guidelines. First, the report should include the precise question posed by the commissioning party as well as the translation, if any, made by the expert to a researchable variant. Second, it should mention all the materials received the expert. This can be important if afterwards, there is confusion about the documents provided to the expert. Third, the expert can be expected to briefly justify why he thinks that he can provide solid advice on the pertinent topic. This can be done by referring to experience with similar reports, scientific publications in the domain, registration as a court expert in the pertinent domain, and/or a resume. Fourth, the expert should briefly summarise the facts of the case, so that it is clear to the reader what these facts are, at least according to the expert. Fifth, the expert should explain in general terms which approach, method is employed to formulate the opinion. As mentioned, it is advisable to employ a method in which alternative hypotheses/scenarios are taken as starting point. The authors further advise peer review as a part of the method. Sixth, there needs to be a short clear conclusion, preferably on how the evidence fits under the alternative hypotheses. In line with the Bayesian view on the position of the expert (Wagenaar, 1988), the authors advise that the expert does not comment on whether the suspect is the perpetrator. Seventh, the expert may want to make short comments about peculiarities detected in the documents, that do not fall within the assignment, if these peculiarities are important to note (obiter dictum). Eighth, reference to relevant literature and appendices, if appropriate, should be included. As examples of relevant appendices, the authors mention detailed information about used tests, or the expert's resume.

References

Ask, K., & Granhag, P. A. (2005). Motivational sources of confirmation bias in criminal investigations: The need for cognitive closure. *Journal of Investigative Psychology and Offender Profiling, 2*, 43–63.

Association of Forensic Science Providers (AFSP). (2009). Standards for the formulation of evaluative forensic science expert opinion. *Science and Justice, 49*, 161–164.

Baron, J., & Hershey, J. C. (1988). Outcome bias in decision evaluation. *Journal of Personality and Social Psychology, 54*, 569–579.

Becker, C. B., Darius, E., & Schaumberg, K. (2007). An analog study of patient preferences for exposure versus alternative treatments for posttraumatic stress disorder. *Behaviour Research and Therapy, 45*, 2861–2873.

Bex, F. J., van Koppen, P. J., Prakken, H., & Verhey, B. (2010). A hybrid formal theory of arguments, stories and criminal evidence. *Artificial Intelligence and Law, 18*, 123–152.

Bowers, K. S., Regehr, G., Balthazard, C., & Parker, K. (1990). Intuition in the context of discovery. *Cognitive Psychology, 22*, 72–110.

Caruso, E. M., Burns, Z. C., & Converse, B. A. (2016). Slow motion increases perceived intent. *Proceedings of the National Academy of Sciences, 113*, 9250–9255.

Cho, K., Barnes, C. M., & Guanara, C. L. (2017). Sleepy punishers are harsh punishers: Daylight saving time and legal sentences. *Psychological Sciences, 28*, 242–247.

Cooper, G. S., & Meterko, V. (2019). Cognitive bias research in forensic science: A systematic review. *Forensic Science International, 297*, 35–46.

Danziger, S., Levav, J., & Avnaim-Pesso, L. (2011). Extraneous factors in judicial decisions. *Proceedings of the National Academy of Sciences, 108*, 6889–6892.

De Keijser, J., & Elffers, H. (2012). Understanding of forensic expert reports by judges, defense lawyers and forensic professionals. *Psychology, Crime and Law, 18*, 191–207.

Douglas, K. S., Lyon, D. R., & Ogloff, J. R. P. (1997). The impact of graphic photographic evidence on mock jurors' decision in a murder trial: Probative of prejudicial? *Law and Human Behavior, 21*, 485–501.

Dror, I. E., Péron, A. E., Hind, S. L., & Charlton, D. (2005). When emotions get the better of us: The effect of contextual top-down processing on matching fingerprints. *Applied Cognitive Psychology, 19*, 799–809.
Dror, I. E., Charlton, D., & Péron, A. E. (2006). Contextual information renders experts vulnerable to making erroneous identifications. *Forensic Science International, 156*, 74–78.
Englich, B., Mussweiler, T., & Strack, F. (2005). The last word in court: A hidden disadvantage for the defense. *Law and Human Behavior, 29*, 705–722.
Englich, B., Mussweiler, T., & Strack, F. (2006). Playing dice with criminal sentences: The influence of irrelevant anchors on experts' judicial decision making. *Personality and Social Psychology Bulletin, 32*, 188–200.
European Network of Forensic Science Institutes (ENFSI). (2016). *Strengthening the evaluation of forensic results across Europe (STEOFRAE)*. https://enfsi.eu
Feigenson, N., & Park, J. (2006). Emotions and attributions of legal responsibility and blame: A research review. *Law and Human Behavior, 30*, 143–161.
Fenton, N., Neil, M., & Lagnado, D. A. (2013). A general structure for legal arguments about evidence using Bayesian networks. *Cognitive Science, 37*, 61–102.
Fenton, N., Neil, M., & Berger, D. (2016). Bayes and the law. *Annual Review of Statistics and its Application, 3*, 51–77.
Findley, K. A., & Scott, M. S. (2006). The multiple dimensions of tunnel vision in criminal cases. *Wisconsin Law Review, 2*, 291–397.
Frederick, S. (2005). Cognitive reflection and decision making. *Journal of Economic Perspectives, 19*, 25–42.
Galton, F. (1892). *Fingerprints*. Macmillan & Co. [2005. New York: Dover publications.].
Gigerenzer, G. (1991). From tools to theories: A heuristic of discovery in cognitive psychology. *Psychological Review, 98*, 254–267.
Goodwin, J. (2000). Wigmore's chart method. *Informal Logic, 20*(3), 223–243.
Greenspan, R., & Scurich, N. (2016). The interdependence of perceived confession voluntariness and case evidence. *Law and Human Behavior, 40*, 650–659.
Gudjonsson, G. H. (1984). A new scale of interrogative suggestibility. *Personality and Individual Differences, 5*, 303–314.
Haack, S. (2003). *Defending science – within reason: Between scientism and cynicism*. Prometheus books.
Hasel, L. E., & Kassin, S. M. (2009). On the presumption of evidentiary independence: Can confessions corrupt eyewitness identifications? *Psychological Science, 20*, 122–126.
Heuer, R. J. (1999). *Psychology of intelligence analyses*. CIA.
Hofvind, S., Skaane, P., Vitak, B., Wang, H., Thoresen, S., Eriksen, L., Bjørndal, H., Braaten, A., & Bjurstam, N. (2005). Influence of review design on percentages of missed interval breast cancers: Retrospective study of interval cancers in a population-based screening program. *Radiology, 237*, 437–443.
Jenkins, G., & Schuller, R. A. (2007). The impact of negative forensic evidence on mock juror's perceptions of a trial of drug-facilitated sexual assault. *Law and Human Behavior, 31*, 369–380.
Johnson-Laird, P. N. (1999). Deductive reasoning. *Annual Review of Psychology, 50*, 109–135.
Kalven, H., & Zeisel, H. (1966). *The American jury*. Little brown.
Kassin, S. M. (1997). The psychology of confession evidence. *American Psychologist, 52*, 221–233.
Kassin, S. M. (2005). On the psychology of confessions: Does innocence put innocents at risk? *American Psychologist, 60*, 215–228.
Kassin, S. M., Dror, I. E., & Kukucka, J. (2013). The forensic confirmation bias: Problems, perspectives, and proposed solutions. *Journal of Applied Research in Memory and Cognition, 2*, 42–52.
Kerstholt, J. H., & Eikelboom, A. R. (2007). Effects of prior interpretation on situation assessment in crime analysis. *Journal of Behavioral Decision Making, 20*, 455–465.

Kerstholt, J. H., & Jackson, J. L. (1998). Judicial decision making: Order of evidence presentation and availability of background information. *Applied Cognitive Psychology, 12*, 445–454.
Kokshoorn, B., Blankers, B. J., de Zoete, J., & Berger, C. E. H. (2017). Activity level DNA evidence evaluation: On propositions addressing the actor of the activity. *Forensic Science International, 278*, 115–124.
Kukucka, J., Kassin, S. M., Zapf, P. A., & Dror, I. E. (2017). Cognitive bias and blindness: A global survey of forensic science examiners. *Journal of Applied Research in Memory and Cognition, 6*, 452–459.
Leclerc, O., Verges, E., & Vial, G. (2022). Turning a graphical method of evidential reasoning into an operational tool for judges? Empirical evidence. *The International Journal of Evidence and Proof, 26*(2), 136–156.
Liebman, J.S., Blackburn, S., Mattern, D., & Waisnor, J. (2012–2013). The evidence of things not seen: Non-matches as evidence of innocence. *Iowa Law Review, 98*, 577–688.
Lilienfeld, S. O., & Landfield, K. (2008). Science and pseudoscience in law enforcement: A user-friendly primer. *Criminal Justice and Behavior, 35*, 1215–1230.
Martire, K. A., Kemp, R. I., Watkins, I., Sayle, M. A., & Newell, B. R. (2013). The expression and interpretation of uncertain forensic science evidence: Verbal equivalence, evidence strength, and the weak evidence effect. *Law and Human Behavior, 37*, 197–207.
McKenzie, C. R. M. (1997). Underweighting alternatives and overconfidence. *Organizational Behavior and Human Decision Processes, 71*, 141–160.
McKenzie, C. R. M. (1998). Taking into account the strength of an alternative hypothesis. *Journal of Experimental Psychology: Learning, Memory, and Cognition, 24*, 771–792.
McKenzie, C. R. M. (1999). (Non)complementary updating of belief in two hypotheses. *Memory & Cognition, 27*, 152–165.
McKenzie, C. R. M., Lee, S. M., & Chen, K. K. (2002). When negative evidence increases confidence: Change in belief after hearing two sides of a dispute. *Journal of Behavioral Decision Making, 15*, 1–18.
Murrie, D. C., Boccaccini, M. T., Guarnera, L. A., & Rufino, K. A. (2013). Are forensic experts biased by the side that retained them? *Psychological Science, 24*, 1889–1897.
Mynatt, C. R., Doherty, M. E., & Dragan, W. (1993). Information relevance, working memory, and the consideration of alternatives. *The Quarterly Journal of Experimental Psychology, 46A*, 759–778.
O'Brien, B. (2009). Prime suspect: An examination of factors that aggravate and counteract confirmation bias in criminal investigations. *Psychology, Public policy, and Law, 15*, 315–334.
Oberlader, V. A., Naefgen, C., Koppehele-Gossel, J., Quinten, L., Banse, R., & Schmidt, A. F. (2016). Validity of content-based techniques to distinguish true and fabricated statements: A meta-analysis. *Law and Human Behavior, 40*, 440–457.
Pacini, R., & Epstein, S. (1999). The relation of rational and experiential information processing styles to personality, basic beliefs, and the ratio-bias phenomenon. *Journal of Personality and Social Psychology, 76*, 972–998.
Pennington, N., & Hastie, R. (1992). Explaining the evidence: Test of the story model for juror decision making. *Journal of Personality and Social Psychology, 62*, 189–206.
Price, R. (1763). An essay towards solving a problem in the doctrine of chances. *Philosophical Transactions of the Royal Society of London, 53*, 370–418.
Rassin, E. (2010). Blindness to alternative scenarios in evidence evaluation. *Journal of Investigative Psychology and Offender Profiling, 7*, 153–163.
Rassin, E. (2013). Presence bias and the insensitivity to the diagnosticity of nonidentifications. *Psychology, Crime & Law, 19*, 203–214.
Rassin, E. (2016). Rational thinking promotes suspect-friendly legal decision making. *Applied Cognitive Psychology, 30*, 460–464.
Rassin, E. (2017a). 'Het is wettig en overtuigend bewezen, althans de kans is 99%': Overwegingen bij het kwantificeren van de strafrechterlijke overtuiging [It is legally and convincingly proven:

That is, the probability is 99%: Considerations about the quantification of legal reasoning]. *Expertise en Recht*, (1), 4–7.
Rassin, E. (2017b). Initial evidence for the assimilation hypothesis. *Psychology, Crime & Law, 23*, 1010–1020.
Rassin, E. (2018a). Fundamental failure to think logically about scientific questions: An illustration of tunnel vision with the application of Wason's Card Selection Test to criminal evidence. *Applied Cognitive Psychology, 32*, 506–511.
Rassin, E. (2018b). Reducing tunnel vision with a pen-and-paper tool for the weighting of criminal evidence. *Journal of Investigative Psychology and Offender Profiling, 15*, 227–233.
Rassin, E. (2020). Context effect and confirmation bias in criminal fact finding. *Legal and Criminological Psychology*. https://doi.org/10.1111/lcrp.12172
Rassin, E., & Israëls, H. (2014). False confessions in the lab: A review. *Erasmus Law Review, 7*, 219–224.
Rassin, E., Eerland, A., & Kuijpers, I. (2010). Let's find the evidence: An analogue study of confirmation bias in criminal investigations. *Journal of Investigative Psychology and Offender Profiling, 7*, 231–246.
Rassin, E., Arbiyah, N., Boskovic, I., Otgaar, H., & Merckelbach, H. (2022). Likelihood ratios in psychological expert opinion, and their reception by professional judges. *International Journal of Evidence and Proof, 26*(4), 325–341.
Richards, P. M., Geiger, J. A., & Tussey, C. M. (2015). The dirty dozen: 12 sources of bias in forensic neuropsychology with ways to mitigate. *Psychological Injury and Law, 8*, 265–280.
Saks, M. J., & Koehler, J. J. (2005). The coming paradigm shift in forensic identification science. *Science, 309*, 892–895.
Simon, D. (2004). A third view of the black box: Cognitive coherence in legal decision making. *The University of Chicago Law Review, 71*, 511–586.
Steblay, N., Dysart, J., Fulero, S., & Lindsay, R. C. L. (2003). Eyewitness accuracy rates in police showup and lineup presentations: A meta-analytic comparison. *Law and Human Behavior, 27*, 523–540.
Steller, M., & Köhnken, G. (1989). Criteria-based statement analysis: Credibility assessment of children's statements in sexual abuse cases. In D. C. Raskin (Ed.), *Psychological methods for investigating evidence* (pp. 217–245). Springer.
Thompson, W. C. (2018). How should forensic scientists present source conclusions? *Seton Hall Law Review, 48*, 773–813.
Thompson, W. C., & Schumann, E. L. (1987). Interpretation of statistical evidence in criminal trials: The prosecutor's fallacy and the defense attorney's fallacy. *Law and Human Behaviour, 11*, 167–187.
Thompson, W. C., Scurrich, N., Dioso-Villa, R., & Velazquez, B. (2017). Evaluating negative forensic evidence: When do jurors treat absence of evidence as evidence of absence? *Journal of Empirical Legal Studies, 14*(3), 569–591.
Thompson, W. C., Vuille, J., Taroni, F., & Biedermann, A. (2018). After uniqueness: The evolution of forensic science. *Judicature, 102*, 18–27.
Van Asch van Wijck, L. H. K. C. (1937). Confrontatie van getuigen met verdachten [Confronting witnesses with suspects]. *Algemeen Nederlandsch Politie-Weekblad voor Rijks- en Gemeentepolitie en de Koninklijke Marechaussee, 22*, 109–111.
Van Koppen, P. J., & Mackor, A. R. (2020). A scenario-approach to the Simonshaven case. *Topics in Cognitive Science, 12*, 1132–1151.
Verhey, B., Bex, F., Timmer, S. J., Vlek, C. S., Meyer, J., Renooij, S., & Prakken, H. (2016). Arguments, scenarios and probabilities: Connections between three normative frameworks for evidential reasoning. *Law, Probability and Risk, 15*, 35–70.
Vredeveldt, A., van Rosmalen, E. A. J., van Koppen, P. J., Dror, I. E., & Otgaar, H. (2022). Legal psychologists as experts: Guidelines for minimizing bias. *Psychology, Crime and Law, 8*(1), 59–75.

Wagenaar, W. A. (1988). The proper seat: A Bayesian discussion of the position of expert witnesses. *Law and Human Behavior, 12*(4), 499–510.

Wagenaar, W. A. (1989). *Identifying Ivan: A case study in legal psychology*. University Press.

Wagenaar, W. A., van Koppen, P. J., & Crombag, H. F. M. (1993). *Anchored narratives: The psychology of criminal evidence*. St. Martin's Press.

Walker, L., & Monahan, J. (1987). Social frameworks: A new use of social science in law. *Virginia Law Review, 73*, 559–598.

Wason, P. C. (1968). Reasoning about a rule. *Quarterly Journal of Experimental Psychology, 20*, 273–281.

Wells, G. L., Bull Kovera, M., Douglass, A. B., Brewer, N., Meissner, C. A., & Wixted, J. T. (2020). Policy and procedure recommendations for the collection and preservation of eyewitness identification evidence. *Law and Human Behavior, 44*, 3–36.

Wigmore, J. H. (1913). *The principles of judicial proof as given by logic, psychology, and general experience, and illustrated in judicial trials*. Little, Brown & Co.

Wilson, J. P., & Rule, N. O. (2015). Facial trustworthiness predicts extreme criminal-sentencing outcome. *Psychological Science, 26*, 1325–1331.

Chapter 2
The Armed Robbery and a Disputed Identification in a Mugshot Series

A tenacious problem for criminal fact finding is that hard facts that help to reconstruct what has happened are oftentimes lacking. In absence of, for example, clear camera footage and undisputed technical evidence, decision makers have to work with witness accounts, on which a story of what happened will be based. Hence, even in the factual account of a case, some degree of interpretation, selection, and even guessing is virtually inevitable.

In this case, it was assumed by the prosecution that two groups of men had joined forces and planned an armed domestic robbery. There was a group of five men referred to as the Bulgarians, and a group of three referred to as the Surinamese. The latter group consisted of coloured individuals. The two groups had not met before, so they did not know each other. It remains unclear how they got in contact, but on March 8, 2010, late at night, they met up in a car parking and decided to rob the pertinent premises. Allegedly, they were convinced that drugs were present on the premises. In the early hours of March 9, at 04:15 h., they forced their way into the house in Roosendaal. The three inhabitants, a 42-year-old woman and her two teenage children, were threatened with a gun and asked about the presumed narcotics. Once it became clear to the robbers that there were no drugs, they took € 45, two watches, a cell phone, and some other small items.

The movements made by the suspect were reconstructed with the accounts of various witnesses who had seen a green car, owned by a friend (E) who was also a suspect in this case. This car with three coloured travellers was seen in Amsterdam on the morning of March 9.

E as well as the five Bulgarians were apprehended swiftly. Our suspect came into the spotlight when the police showed the Bulgarians ten pictures of men, who were possible coperpetrators of E. It is not completely clear how the police selected these pictures. Probably because they were all ex-convicts from the same network as E. It appears that they even showed pictures of the arrested suspects to each other (i.e.,

ECLI:NL:GHAMS:2012:BV2834.

E. Rassin, *Case Studies in Legal Psychology*,
https://doi.org/10.1007/978-3-031-44931-4_2

suspects were even shown pictures of themselves). The police wrote in their file that four of the five Bulgarians identified the suspect as one of the three coperpetrators. Unfortunately, the documents were not detailed. There was no information on the selection of the pictures, the instructions given to the Bulgarians, the order of exposure, whether the Bulgarians had contact with each other, or whether other people were also identified during these procedures. The defence lawyer asked me for an opinion on the identification of the suspect by the four Bulgarians.

2.1 Varieties of Identification Procedures

In this case, the police took ten pictures of potential suspects from their files and showed these to five witnesses/suspects. Obviously, there are other ways of setting up an eyewitness identification procedure. It is important to note that procedures differ as to their purpose and quality standards. In the current case, the police were convinced that there were more perpetrators than the six suspects (five Bulgarians plus E) already arrested. The purpose of the identification procedure was to find the seventh (and eighth?) perpetrator. Hence, the priority was to establish reasonable cause of suspicion against a yet unknown suspect. Framed in the opposite way: The worst possible mistake in this instance is that the police cannot find the seventh and eighth perpetrator. Friedrich (1993) argued that decision makers strive not always to reach the best conclusion, but sometimes merely to avoid the worst possible outcome. He speaks of a primary error detection and minimisation (in short: PEDMIN). Given that the sole purpose of the identification procedure was to find additional suspects, the emphasis was on finding these suspects, but not on creating the highest quality evidence against the suspects. By contrast, if the police already have their suspect, the emphasis will be on creating evidence that will do well in court. An identification procedure aimed at creating evidence ideally prioritises high quality. In this case, PEDMIN dictates that a positive identification should not be false, because that may contribute to a miscarriage of justice. Consequently, quality demands will be raised. In sum, the purpose of the identification procedure may partly determine its content and form, and eventually the strength of a positive identification, if any.

Regardless of its purpose, an identification procedure can take the form of a live confrontation, a photo confrontation, or a video variant. All variants have their advantages. For example, in live and video procedures, dynamics can be incorporated (e.g., have the individual(s) make certain movements or sounds). While a photo procedure is by definition static, it is much easier to carry out than a live procedure. With photos it is also quite easy to zoom in on faces. In all, there seems to be no general effect of presentation modus on patterns of outcomes (Wells et al., 2020).

Another source of differences is whether the witness is shown to just one person (a show up) or multiple (e.g., a mugshot series or a line-up). Particularly for procedures that aim at creating evidence against the known suspect, multiple procedures are recommendable (e.g., Wells et al., 2020). If a multiple procedure is chosen, there is one more differentiation, namely whether all individuals will be shown simultaneously or sequentially to the witness (Steblay et al., 2011).

2.2 Estimator Variables

The variants of identification procedures discussed in the previous paragraph are largely under the control of the police. That is, the police determine the purpose, content, and form of the procedures. These procedural variants are hence known as system variables. However, there are also numerous factors that may affect the witnesses' performance that are not under the control of the police, simply because they occur outside of their influence. Those factors are referred to as estimator variables. Some of these variables concern the witness. For example, it has been argued that people differ in their ability to perceive and recognize other people's faces. Perfect et al. (2007) found that people with a preference for global visual processing, as opposed to local or detailed processing, are slightly better at identifying others. Besides such trait-like characteristics of the witness, their state during witnessing can also affect the performance in a subsequent identification procedure. For example, perceived stress may suppress identification performance. Imagine that a victim of robbery is asked later to identify the suspect in a police identification procedure. It turns out that if the perpetrator threatened the victim with a weapon, the victim will be less accurate in his attempt to recognize the suspect. This is due to the automatic concentration on the strongest emotion eliciting stimulus (namely the weapon), resulting in inferior observation of the perpetrator's facial appearance, inhibiting later recognition. In a meta-analysis, Steblay (1992) found that this so-called weapon focus effect is stronger for guns than for meat cleavers. The magnitude of the effect was not affected by the retention interval between the crime and the identification procedure. Finally, it seems that the presence of a weapon primarily reduces the capacity to recognize the perpetrator, but it may also lead to innocent fillers being falsely identified more readily.

While witness characteristics may affect the outcome of the identification procedure, this may also hold for perpetrator characteristics. One can imagine that very distinctive features of the perpetrator's face may facilitate identification (Wagenaar, 1989). There may also be an interaction between witness and perpetrator, in that identification is facilitated if both belong to the same race or even culture. People have some difficulty distinguishing individuals from other races, which is referred to as crossracial insensitivity (Wells et al., 2020).

Finally, various situation characteristics may affect identification outcome. For example, exposure time seems to be correlated with identification performance (e.g., Wagenaar, 1989). Wagenaar and van der Schrier (1996) tested the effect of illumination level and distance during witnessing, on the accuracy of identification in a subsequent well-conducted evidentiary line-up (see Chap. 3 for a discussion of line-ups). They showed a picture of an unfamiliar person to 56 undergraduates,

Table 2.1 True (bold) and false positive likelihoods (Wagenaar & van der Schrier, 1996)

	Illumination level (lux)								
Distance (m)	0.3	2	3	5	10	30	150	300	3000
3	**14** 9	**46** 10	**61** 8	**79** 8	**82** 6	**82** 6	**82** 3	**86** 2	**86** 2
5	**11** 5	**25** 11	**54** 5	**50** 1	**68** 1	**79** 1	**82** 0	**86** 0	**86** 1
7		**7** 5	**36** 9	**43** 6	**71** 5	**68** 5	**82** 3	**79** 2	**86** 1
12			**4** 4	**25** 6	**43** 4	**43** 4	**57** 1	**57** 1	**61** 1
20				**11** 5	**18** 9	**18** 9	**43** 8	**39** 8	**57** 5
30					**14** 4	**25** 7	**21** 6	**32** 6	**36** 6
40						**7** 3	**14** 8	**25** 8	**29** 9

under different levels of illumination and distance. Subsequently, the participants underwent a photo line-up procedure including six pictures (some of which were target-present, others target-absent). Outcomes of the line-up procedures are presented in Table 2.1. As can be seen, illumination and distance had a strong effect on identification accuracy. The authors postulated the rule of 15: For a valid identification with a likelihood ratio of at least 15, while witnessing the crime, the witness should be no further away than 15 m, and illumination should be no less than 15 lux.

As mentioned, the police have no influence on estimator variables. Nonetheless, these factors can affect identification accuracy. Therefore, the police should at least do their best to address all potentially relevant estimator variables in a pre-line up interview and to document these carefully (Wells et al., 2020).

2.3 How This Case Ended

The absence of good police documentation makes it difficult to determine precisely what the police did in this case. What is clear is that they showed ten pictures to the five Bulgarian suspects. The defence lawyer showed me the pictures. There were seven pictures of Caucasian men and three of dark coloured men. It seems that the police simply collected pictures of their arrested suspects and a few additional potential suspects based on the initial information provided by witnesses. Our suspect belonged to the latter group, because witnesses had seen him in the early morning of March 9 in Amsterdam in the green car together with E. Hypothesis was that they had committed the crime together and went back home to Amsterdam afterwards. It may seem strange that the police showed photographs of their suspects to the suspects themselves, but obviously they were trying to find the complete group of perpetrators. Because four of the five suspects testified that our suspect was involved, he was incriminated. However, if these four identifications are subsequently not only used as a starting point for further investigation, but also as evidence, their strength may not be as great as it seems at first sight. Admittedly, if the four positive identifications had been made in well-conducted evidence line-ups, it would have been all too coincidental that the suspect was identified four times. The likelihood of that happening by chance would be 0.10^4. However, the present procedure fell short of an evidence line-up in several ways (see Chap. 3 for line-up standards). For example, in a line-up, there is just one suspect, with at least five known innocent foils selected because of their match with the description of the perpetrator, and all this is communicated to the witness. In this case, all pictures were of suspects, and they were not selected based on their resemblance with a description of the perpetrator. Further, for the four identifications to be construed as strong evidence, they have to be made independently from each other. It was unclear whether this was so. Perhaps, all five Bulgarians sat in the same room at the same time, and were all shown the pictures. Also, the instruction was unknown. Arguably, the question of whether the suspect recognizes anyone from the set of pictures as occasional partner in this crime will yield fewer identifications than the instruction that 'we know that all these people were involved, so you had better confirms that'.

If we assume the worst, the four identifications provide little evidence at all. Even if we trust that the mugshots were accompanied by correct, conservative instructions, and all suspects went through the procedure individually and independently, the evidentiary power of the identifications in this multiple mugshot series is limited. In essence, the witness undergoes a show up repeatedly. For every picture, the witness has to decide whether or not the person is familiar. Quite generally, the likelihood of a true identification in a show up is about 47%, and that of a false positive 23% (see Steblay et al., 2003, for an overview). Hence, the combined strength of four identifications can be estimated at (47% / 23% =) 2^4, equals 16. In hindsight, the strength of the evidence could have been increased if the police had subjected one of the suspects to their improvised mugshot series and, after an initial identification of this suspect, had set up good line-ups for the remaining three witnesses/suspects. The positive identification by these three, if any, in a good line-up would have had much more strength.

In my report for the defence, I wrote that the identifications served well as a starting point for further investigations against the suspect, but they fell short as evidence. Several factors suppressed the validity of the identifications. First, the procedure was a mugshot series during which witnesses were asked to identify multiple suspects from a set of ten pictures. This context may foster false identifications. Second, the perpetrators had met under suboptimal conditions, particularly because it was dark. Third, for the Bulgarians, there may have been a crossracial insensitivity at play. Finally, the identifications could not be said to have been made independently. Rather, there were some indications that the suspects made their identifications in each other's presence. For the last argument, I referred to an article by Hasel and Kassin (2009), as an example of a paper about the importance of evidentiary independence.

The court did use the four identifications as evidence, along with the fact that the suspect had kept silent for the most part of the investigation, and finally gave an account that was not verifiable, and the evidence suggesting that the suspect was in the company of E (who had been convicted for this crime) in the hours following this robbery. With regard to my report, the court argued that they agreed that positive identifications resulting from show ups should be interpreted with caution. That was why the court did not see the identification in isolation, but in combination with the other evidence. The court found the comment about suboptimal witnessing circumstances and crossracial insensitivity speculative. They did not see why the findings from one single study (i.e., Hasel & Kassin, 2009) should affect their decision. Finally, they did not perceive any information suggesting that the identifications were false. The suspect was convicted to 5 years imprisonment.

References

Friedrich, J. (1993). Primary error detection and minimization (PEDMIN) strategies in social cognition: A reinterpretation of confirmation bias phenomena. *Psychological Review, 100*, 298–319.

Hasel, L. E., & Kassin, S. M. (2009). On the presumption of evidentiary independence: Can confessions corrupt eyewitness identifications? *Psychological Science, 20*, 122–126.

Perfect, T. J., Dennis, I., & Snell, A. (2007). The effects of local and global processing orientation on eyewitness identification performance. *Memory, 15*, 784–798.

Steblay, N. M. (1992). A meta-analytic review of the weapon focus effect. *Law and Human Behavior, 16*, 413–424.

Steblay, N., Dysart, J., Fulero, S., & Lindsay, R. C. L. (2003). Eyewitness accuracy rates in police showup and lineup presentations: A meta-analytic comparison. *Law and Human Behavior, 27*, 523–540.

Steblay, N. K., Dysart, J. E., & Wells, G. L. (2011). Seventy-two tests of the sequential lineup superiority effect: A meta-analysis and policy discussion. *Psychology, Public Policy, and Law, 17*, 99–139.

Wagenaar, W. A. (1989). *Identifying Ivan: A case study in legal psychology*. University Press.

Wagenaar, W. A., & van der Schrier, J. H. (1996). Face recognition as a function of distance and illumination: A practical tool for use in the courtroom. *Psychology, Crime & Law, 2*, 321–332.

Wells, G. L., Bull Kovera, M., Douglass, A. B., Brewer, N., Meissner, C. A., & Wixted, J. T. (2020). Policy and procedure recommendations for the collection and preservation of eyewitness identification evidence. *Law and Human Behavior, 44*, 3–36.

Chapter 3
The Armed Robbery and a Disputed Identification in a Line Up

One evening in November 2012, a middle-aged woman answers the doorbell. Two men force their way in and threaten her with physical violence. Her son is also threatened. After some time, the robbers leave with approximately € 10,000. The victim calls the police. During the investigation of the crime scene, the police find remains of a cigarette. With the DNA secured from this cigarette, the police find a suspect. Two years later, in August 2014, the woman and her son are subjected to a computerised sequential line up. The woman does not identify anyone, but her son does point out the suspect. He also testifies that he has seen the suspect once after the incident. The suspect denies. He claims to have visited his girlfriend on the pertinent evening to celebrate her son's birthday. The girlfriend confirms this alibi under oath. He does not deny that he may have smoked a cigarette in the neighbourhood of the robbery because he had visited the area as a door-to-door salesman at that time. The suspect was convicted to 30 months imprisonment. During appeal, I was asked to give advice on the strength of the identification. No one was ever arrested as the second robber.

3.1 Fifty Rules for a Proper Line Up Identification Procedure

In this instance, the police set up an evidence line up for the victims. The main idea behind the evidence line up is that a positive identification, if any, can only be attributed to one thing, namely that the witness indeed must have seen the suspect commit the crime. For this idea to be reasonable, and hence for the identification to be construed as strong evidence, many factors have to be in place. In 1989, Wagenaar wrote an extensive overview of characteristics that make an evidence line up

---

ECLI:NL:GHDHA:2017:536

E. Rassin, *Case Studies in Legal Psychology*,
https://doi.org/10.1007/978-3-031-44931-4_3

actually a good line up. There is an impressive history to Wagenaar's (1989) book. In 1976, a Ukrainian immigrant in the United States John Demjanjuk was recognised in the street by a WW II concentration camp survivor as Ivan the terrible. Ivan the Terrible was a war criminal who was responsible for the death of 850,000 prisoners in concentration camp Treblinka, in 1942–1943. Particularly, he gassed these victims with exhaust fumes from a tank. He was also notoriously cruel. In 1987, Demjanjuk was tried for these war crimes. Dutch professor of psychology, Dr. Willem Albert Wagenaar served as an expert witness and gave his opinion on the quality of the identifications in this case. Later, he wrote a book about the case, in which he presented no less than 50 rules for the proper administration of a line up procedure (Wagenaar, 1989). Some of these rules are more crucial to the validity of an identification than others. Further, by now, some rules may appear to be old fashioned, outdated, caught up by new insights and modern technologies. Notwithstanding, the 50 rules offer a good insight in the rationale behind the line up procedure. They seek to optimise the system variables of the identification, that is, all variables that affect the validity of the identification and that are under the control of the justice system. Below, the 50 rules are discussed.

1. *If the witness knew the suspect prior to the crime, an identification procedure is not in place as evidence.* It should be acknowledged that it construes evidence if the witness who does not know the suspect picks this suspect from a line up. If the line up procedure follows all rules that follow, such a positive identification can virtually only be explained if the suspect is indeed the perpetrator. Therein lies the evidentiary strength. However, if the witness already knew the perpetrator, it suffices that he points him out to the police. Conducting a line up is, in this situation, superfluous. It may even construe fake evidence because it is obvious that we are able to pick someone we know well from a line up of similar individuals. In this instance, the police should gather evidence other than identification evidence delivered by this witness.
2. *If an identification is to be used as evidence, the witness should be subjected to a line up, not to a show up procedure.* If the police have a witness who saw the perpetrator, and did not know him beforehand, an identification procedure can be set up to yield evidence to be used in the trial later on. The police can then choose between a show up and a line up. Obviously, a show up is easier to conduct because in the line up, several foils will have to be selected and included. Psychologically, however, a line up can be expected to yield stronger evidence than a show up. This is so because a positive identification in a show up can be attributed more readily to alternative causes, that is, other causes than that the suspect is the perpetrator. For example, even if the witness is not quite certain, he might still testify that he recognises the person (photo) to which he is exposed, merely because the shown individual resembles his recollection of the perpetrator somewhat, or because he reckons that the police will not show this person if it were not the perpetrator, or even because the witness would not want to disappoint the police by testifying that he does not recognise the suspect. All these alternative causes are actually potential causes of a false positive

identification. In theory, these alternative reasons for a positive identification are ruled out in a line up procedure, simply because the witness is exposed to several individuals from which he has to select the perpetrator. Hence, while in a show up procedure, the witness can suffice with replying "yes" to the question whether he recognises the suspect; this answer is not even in place in a line up procedure, where the crucial question is not whether the witness recognises the suspect (no/yes), but whether any of the shown individuals is the perpetrator (i.e., which number, if any). Thus, in a sense, the line up procedure asks more from the witness than does the show up. All this is so to exclude alternative explanations for a positive identification and, hence, to prevent false positive identifications. The theoretical superiority of the line up versus the show up has been studied several times. Note that superiority can be construed differently depending on the angle one has. From a legal psychological stance, superiority refers to the accuracy of the evidence. That is, evidence is superior if it does not suffer false positives. From an investigative psychological stance (i.e., employing psychological insights to gather more evidence), however, superiority may also be defined by the likelihood of producing evidence against the suspect. Consequently, a procedure that solely yields negative outcomes is superior to the legal psychologist, but not to the investigative psychologist. Steblay et al. (2003) wrote a meta-analysis of eight papers on the strength of show ups and line ups. Their work illustrates that it can be quite complex to compare the two procedures, in part because different definitions of superiority can be taken as starting point. They conclude firstly that, in case of a target-present display (i.e., the perpetrator is present in the line up, or the police have the right suspect in the show up), the likelihood of a correct positive identification is about 47% in the show up and 45% in the line up procedure. In the target-absent displays (i.e., the perpetrator is absent from the line up, or the police have the wrong suspect in the show up), the likelihood of a false positive identification is 23% in the show up and 17% in the line up. These numbers appear to differ little. However, when calculating likelihood ratios, the overall likelihood ratio for an identification in a show up turns out to be (47%: 23% =) 2, while that for an identification in a line up is (45%: 17% =) 2.7 = > 3. Hence, the line up is indeed superior in this sense. At the same time, the show ups yielded an overall correct decision outcome of 69% compared to only 51% for the line ups. This is so because line ups make the witness more conservative and reluctant to make a positive identification. Further, the line up yields the possibility to identify a foil, which is an incorrect outcome that is, however, not detrimental to accuracy in that it will not construe evidence against the suspect. It will merely display that the witness must be mistaken. Obviously, selecting a foil (i.e., a mistake unfortunate for the witness, but not detrimental to accuracy) is impossible in case of show ups because these lack foils. Wagenaar (1989) was quite pronounced in his preference for line ups compared to show ups. He argued that if the goal of the procedure is to produce evidence against the known suspect, the police should only conduct a line up, never a show up. For him, an evidence identification procedure is by definition a line up. Of course, legal systems are not bound by

Wagenaar's or any other scientists' insights, and in many systems, show up identifications, and even identifications aimed at finding a suspect, are considered as evidence in criminal procedures.

3. *An identification based on a procedure merely including mugshots should not be used as evidence.* If the police have a database including many suspects, it might be tempting to use photographs of these suspects as foils in an ongoing investigation. Obviously, it is much easier to select photos matching the perpetrator's description from a mugshot database, compared to a database of random people because the average person will not voluntarily give his photo to the police to be used in line ups. However, for a line up procedure to be optimally valid, the foils should be positively innocent. This may not be the case for ex-suspects whose photos are used in a line up (unless they are dead, incarcerated, or have a watertight alibi). Moreover, not only should the foils be innocent, the witness needs to be informed that the line up consists of the suspect and innocent foils. This is not to needlessly stress the witness, but to make him conservative, and ultimately to raise the bar for a positive identification, simultaneously suppressing the likelihood of a false positive.
4. *If a witness was confronted with mugshots, he should not be subjected to another identification procedure later on.* This guideline, and several others that will follow, aims to prevent a positive identification in the line up that is actually caused by the witness recognising the suspect not from the crime per se but from the previous identification procedure (cf. a false fame effect; Jacoby et al., 1989, or bystander effect, which originally refers to mistakenly recognising a bystander as the perpetrator). Imagine that a witness claims to recognise a photo during the confrontation with mugshots. If the police organise a line up later on, and the witness again identifies the same suspect, this does actually not add anything to the original identification in the mugshot exposure session. This line up really only tests whether the witness at the time of the line up remembers who he identified during the mugshot series. A positive identification during the line up may, thus, well be due to the witness remembering the suspect from the mugshots rather than from the crime. Even if this source monitoring error is absent, the witness might simply feel committed to identifying the suspect again, out of a need to be consistent with his previous choice. Or finally, the witness may notice that the suspect is the only person who appeared in both identification procedures, which implies that he must indeed be the suspect.
5. *If a line up is possible and in place, it is preferable over a mugshot procedure.* As implied in rule four, it must be acknowledged that once exposed to the suspect in any identification procedure, the witness is no longer usable in later procedures. This means that the police have to consider carefully what they want from their witness(es). If they decide to use the witness to apprehend a suspect via confrontation to a mugshot series, they cannot use the witness later on to provide evidence against this suspect. Wagenaar (1989) would advise to seek and use other means to find the suspect, and to save the witness for a line up. The idea behind this advice is that it is generally harder to find strong evidence than to gather information that leads to the apprehension of a suspect.

6. *If the suspect was apprehended* via *a mugshot identification, the subsequent identification in an otherwise flawless line up procedure has suppressed evidentiary power*. If the suspect is apprehended via a mugshot identification, the case against him starts with his facial appearance. Obviously, identifications in line up procedures also revolve around facial appearances. Hence, the evidence then heavily leans on the similarity in appearance between the suspect and the perpetrator. If there were to be an anomaly such that the innocent suspect has a remarkable similarity with the perpetrator, leaning on identification both for apprehension of the suspect and for the evidence against him becomes risky.
7. *A witness should not undergo more than one identification procedure targeting one suspect*. This rule is a broader variant of rule number four. It seeks to prevent a cross-over effect, particularly the false fame effect.
8. *Identification evidence in absence of another kind of evidence does not suffice to convict the suspect*. This rule follows the same logic as rule number six. That is, there is always a chance that an anomaly in the appearance of the perpetrator and/or the suspect fuels false positive identifications. Therefore, it is advisable to combine identification evidence with other kinds of evidence.
9. *Identification evidence always needs to be accompanied by other evidence, not identification evidence*. This rule is a positively phrased version of rule eight.
10. *If there is more than one witness, police should strive to use the remaining witnesses to falsify an initial identification*. With this rule, Wagenaar (1989) seeks to introduce scientific thinking in the domain of identification evidence. The rule dictates that an initial identification should be followed by new identifications in which it becomes even less likely that the suspect be identified falsely. This can be achieved by eliciting detailed descriptions of the perpetrator and matching the foils closely.
11. *All identification attempts, whether success or failure, have to be written down in the report*. One can imagine that if a witness does not identify the suspect, the police will not make up a report of this failed attempt, merely because the nonidentification does not add to the evidence against the suspect. However, in recent decades, in the literature, the insight has emerged that negative evidence, such as a nonidentification, can actually be diagnostic of the suspect's innocence. Therefore, nonidentifications have to be reported. Wells and Lindsay (1980) reanalysed data from a study by Loftus (1976) and noticed that in case of culprit-present procedures, 84% of the witnesses identified him, while 16% did not. In case of culprit-absent line ups, 60% identified the innocent suspect (who was a bystander) and 40% made a nonidentification. Assuming equal base rate, this pattern of results may well indicate that of all identifications, 58% (i.e., 84 out of 144) are correct. Also, out of 56 nonidentifications, 71% indicate that the suspect is in fact innocent. These considerations underline the importance of nonidentifications. They even suggest that nonidentifications are more diagnostic of innocence, than identifications are of guilt. Hence, the authors concluded that "there is no justifiable logic for approaching a lineup procedure with a set for considering an identification of the suspect to be informative

while considering a nonidentification to be uninformative" (Wells & Lindsay, 1980, p. 777).

While the argument of Wells and Lindsay (1980) is theoretical, and supported by only one empirical study in which the innocent suspect was a bystander, the previously discussed meta-analysis by Steblay et al. (2003) suggests that target-absent show ups lead in 85% of the cases to a nonidentification, as do 53% of the target-present show ups. Hence, these findings confirm that nonidentifications are diagnostic of innocence in show ups. For the line ups, target-absent line ups resulted in 57% of the cases in nonidentifications, while target-present line ups yielded 55% misses. This suggests that nonidentifications in line ups are hardly diagnostic. In a larger scale meta-analysis, Clark et al. (2008) included 94 experiments on line up accuracy. In the culprit-present line ups, the culprit was identified in 46% of the cases, while in 21% the eyewitness identified a foil, and in 33% no identification was made. In case of culprit-absent procedures, 13% falsely identified the innocent suspect, 35% identified a foil, and 52% made no identification. Controlling for sample sizes, the authors computed the following likelihood ratios. A positive identification turned out to be 5.4 times likelier if the suspect is guilty than if he is innocent. An identification of a foil is 2.0 times likelier in case of innocence compared to guilt. Finally, a nonidentification is 2.1 times likelier in case of innocence compared to guilt. Hence, the data support the diagnostic power of suspect identifications for guilt, but also the exonerating diagnostic power of foil identifications and line up rejections. In conclusion, the outcome of a line up procedure is not only interesting if the suspect is identified by the eyewitness. Should the witness fail to identify anyone (i.e., a nonidentification or complete rejection of the line up), this indicates that the suspect may be innocent. The same can be said about the identification of a foil. Using Bayesian analyses, Wells and Olson (2002) argue that 'the exonerating value of filler identification and "not there" responses can actually exceed the incriminating value of identifications of the suspect' (p. 155). So, whereas it is not clear exactly how diagnostic foil identifications and nonidentifications are of the suspect's innocence, it seems fair to conclude that both outcomes have at least considerable diagnostic value. Therefore, nonidentifications are crucial to the defence, but also to the judge (and jury), in order to correctly estimate the probability of guilt. In spite of the importance of nonidentifications, Wells and Lindsay (1980) argued that 'neither jurors and judges nor police investigators place much faith in the eyewitness who says "this is not the man"' (p. 776). As to the diagnostic power of foil identifications, Clark and Wells (2008) argue that it may be 'particularly easy for the casual observer to dismiss the diagnostic value of foil identifications because they are known immediately to be mistaken identifications; the eyewitness has made a mistake so the witness must have a bad memory. At one level this is true – the witness has made a mistake. But the nature of the mistake suggests that the eyewitness is saying "Your suspect in this lineup looks less like the perpetrator than does this foil," which should logically reduce the fact-finder's confidence that the suspect is the perpetrator' (p. 419).

12. *Reports of failed identification attempts should include all information necessary to interpret the failure*. Intuitively, a nonidentification may quite readily be explained away (Rassin, 2013). However, as discussed under the previous rule, nonidentifications may be diagnostic of the suspect's innocent. Hence, it is important to discuss possible reasons for the nonidentification, and therefore, information that can shed light on these causes should be documented.
13. *Subsequent identifications have less evidentiary power than does the initial identification*. Possibly, the police start from nothing when setting up a line up. Even if they do their utmost to build a bias-free line up, completely excluding bias is difficult. Hence, if there is a bias in the line up, and the police use this biased line up for more than one witness, the bias will be carried over to all subsequent witness identifications.
14. *If there are more than one witness, they should be prevented from having contact*. Preventing contact between witnesses is important because during contact, a witness who already underwent the line up procedure may give advice to another witness who has yet to do the line up. For example, the former witness may inform the latter witness that he identified number two in the line up and that the police officer said that number two was indeed the suspect. If this were to happen, a positive identification by the second witness has no evidentiary power, even though it may well be treated as evidence nonetheless.
15. *If the witness discussed the case with others, prior to the identification procedure, this should be documented in the report*. A witness may have talked to other witnesses (or other third parties), and during such conversations, the witness may have been influenced. For example, the facial appearance of the perpetrator may have been discussed, and this discussion may have altered the witness' recollection of the perpetrator.
16. *If a witness is expected to be able to successfully identify the suspect due to information he received from third parties, he should be excluded from the procedure*. This rule is a consequence of rule number 15. If a witness is able to identify the suspect due to information received from others instead of his own perception, the possible positive identification has no real evidentiary power.
17. *Prior to undergoing an identification procedure, the witness needs to produce a verbal description of the perpetrator. This description has to be included in the report*. It is important to acknowledge that all evidence suffers imperfection. Against this background, imagine a witness who has actually not seen the perpetrator very well. If this witness is subjected to a line up containing six individuals (one suspect and five foils), there is a one in six probability (17%) that he accidentally points out the suspect. To prevent such 'bad' witnesses (or better: nonwitnesses) from being in a line up procedure, it is advisable to only include witnesses who are able to give a sensible verbal description of the perpetrator. Note that producing a verbal description is quite difficult because facial appearance is difficult to grasp in words. Producing a verbal description of the perpetrator's face may even affect the witness' recollection of that face, due to the verbal labelling effect (Carmichael et al., 1932). Meissner and Brigham (2001) conducted a meta-analysis of 15 publications on the effect of

giving a verbal description on subsequent identification accuracy. Overall, giving a verbal description indeed slightly suppressed identification accuracy (Fisher's $Z_r = -0.12$). The authors also found that the verbal labelling effect was more prominent if the identification procedure takes place immediately after giving the verbal description (i.e., <10 min), but virtually disappears if the procedure takes place after a delay of more than 30 minutes. In conclusion, having the witness give a verbal description of the perpetrator seeks to prevent that non-witnesses accidentally falsely identify the suspect, but simultaneously suppresses the witnesses' capacity to identify the suspect.

18. *A witness whose verbal description of the perpetrator does not match the suspect should be excluded from the procedure.* Obviously, if the witness' verbal description of the perpetrator does not match the appearance of the suspect, there must be something wrong. Either the witness is mistaken, or the suspect is not the perpetrator. In this situation, conducting a line up seems senseless, and may well be dangerous due to the statistical likelihood of an accidental false identification.
19. *The witness needs to be instructed that he is allowed to point out just one person in the line up, and that this person should fit the description given by the witness.* Say, there are six individuals in the line up, and thus the statistical chance of an accidental identification of the suspect is one in six (17%) or even one in seven (14%) including the option of rejecting the complete line up. This known and relatively modest false positive likelihood will decrease even more with increasing numbers of foils. However, if the witness is allowed to identify more than one individual as possible perpetrators, the likelihood of an accidental selection of the suspect increases. Hence, the present rule aims to suppress the likelihood of a false identification, as do most of Wagenaar's (1989) rules. Obviously, if all other rules presented by Wagenaar ad adhered to, all people in the line up should fit the witness' description of the perpetrator.
20. *The instruction given to the witness has to be included literally in the report.* The instruction given to the witness is a crucial part of the line up procedure. It has to include several warnings (e.g., that the perpetrator may not be in the line up, that the witness should only identify an individual if he is quite confident, that all foils are known to be innocent, that indeed only one individual (at most) is to be identified) and simultaneously has to be free from suggestion (e.g., manipulating the witness into identifying a particular individual, or even to make a positive identification, anyway). It is important to verify that the proper instruction was given to the witness, and therefore, the instruction has to be documented.
21. *The witness should be instructed that the perpetrator may not be in the line up, and that therefore, he should only identify someone if he is confident.* It is possible that the witness experiences unspoken pressure to identify someone from the line up. To relieve this pressure, the witness should be informed that he need not necessarily make a positive identification. After all, it is possible that the suspect is innocent, and is therefore not recognised by the witness.

22. *The police officer supervising the identification procedure should be knowledgeable about identification evidence.* Given that there are many rules and guidelines for the correct execution of an identification procedure, it is obviously important that the supervising police officer makes no mistakes that can ruin the evidentiary power of the outcome.
23. *A line up should never include more than one suspect.* There is a straightforward statistical rational for the line up procedure, namely that if there are six individuals in the line up, the statistical baseline probability of a false positive is one in six (17%). Obviously, if more than one suspect were to be included in the line up, without increasing the number of foils, this statistical argument is ruined.
24. *The witness should be informed that there is only one suspect in the line up. If the witness has stated that he saw more than one perpetrator, he needs to be clear about which perpetrator the line up is targeting.* It is possible that a witness witnessed a multiperpetrator crime. Obviously, for each suspect a separate line up has to be set up, each with matching foils. Ultimately, it must be clear to the witness which suspect a particular line up is targeting.
25. *If a witness saw more than one perpetrator, there should be a separate line up for each suspect. A foil can only act in one of these line ups.* Building on the previous rule, it must be understood that each line up has to include separate foils. If a foil can theoretically serve in two separate line ups, because he matches the descriptions of both perpetrators, he should still be included in only one. Otherwise, the witness, when participating in the second line up, will consider that the pertinent foil must indeed be a foil because he was in the first line up as well. In this situation, the foil is no longer a serious foil in the second line up.
26. *The witness has to be informed that he is allowed to point out just one person from the line up.* This rule is merely a reiteration of rule number 19.
27. *In a line up, there should at least be 6 individuals, preferably 10 through 12.* Taking the baseline statistical starting point mentioned above, that is, the chance level probability of picking the suspect if there are 5 foils is 1 in 6 (17%), an increase in foils will reduce the theoretical chance of a false positive to 14% with 6 foils, 12.5% with 7 foils, 11% with 8 foils, 10% with 9 foils, 9% with 10 foils, and 8% with 11 foils. These likelihoods ignore the option of a complete rejection of the line up. Thus, the more foils, the "better" the line up. Obviously, however, there is a law of diminishing returns and ultimately a ceiling effect, and Wagenaar (1989) argues that increases in foil numbers exceeding 11 no longer decrease the likelihood of a false positive, while increasing difficulties with setting up the large line up. Hence, the optimal number of foils is around 11. At the bottom end, Wagenaar notes that the literature does not resist line ups with five or more foils. Hence, he argued that the minimum number of foils can be set at five.
28. *All foils should fit the verbal description of the perpetrator given by the witness.* By now, this rule may be perceived as obvious. The evidentiary strength of a positive identification in a line up procedure largely rests on the idea that the

witness was able to pick the suspect from a pool of individuals who all might have been the perpetrator (i.e., appearance-wise). Notably, this is only true if all foils look like the suspect as far as the suspect and all foils match the description.

29. *If the suspect does not match the description of the perpetrator given by the witness, that description cannot be used to select foils*. Obviously, if the suspect markedly does not match the description of the perpetrator, there is something wrong. In this case, a line up should not be considered (see rule 30 below). More prudently, if the suspect does not match the description, but all foils do, the suspect will end up standing out from the others in the line up, making the line up biased.
30. *If there is no verbal description of the perpetrator available that matches the suspect, a line up becomes difficult or even impossible*. Related to, and more conservatively than the previous rule, if the suspect does not match the description of the perpetrator, something is wrong, and a line up should not be considered.
31. *Foils should not stem from a homogeneous group, such as police officers*. If all foils stem from the same homogeneous group, there is a risk of a subtle commonality between the foils that lack in the suspect. For example, if all foils wear the same military boots, whereas the suspect does not, this makes the suspect stand out, thus making the line up unfair.
32. *Mock witnesses* (i.e., *individuals who were not witnesses to the crime, but are given the description of the perpetrator and are subjected to the line up procedure) should not be able to pick the suspect*. If there are six people in the line up, the suspect should not be picked more often than one-sixth of the times by these mock witnesses. If the suspect is picked significantly more often than chance level, this suggests that the line up is somehow biased (see Tredoux, 1998). The problem of biased line ups was originally addressed by Doob and Kirshenbaum (1973). Hence, a mock witness test is sometimes referred to as a Doob and Kirshenbaum test. Although conducting a Doob and Kirshenbaum test is quite a lot of extra work, it is probably the best way to ensure that the line up is unbiased and fair.
33. *It should be impossible to discover that a foil cannot be the suspect*. Again, the idea is that a positive identification in a line up procedure has strong evidentiary power because the witness picked the suspect from a line up of at least six possible individuals. This idea is ruined if the witness knows that some of the individuals included in the line up can actually not be the suspect. This may be so if the witness just saw one or several police officers in the hall way, who are now included in the line up. Obviously, the statistical likelihood that the witness will then identify the suspect inflates. Note that errors like this may remain hidden from sight, resulting in an unjustified belief in the positive identification.
34. *If the line up is carried out with photos, the photos should be retained, together with the position in which they were shown simultaneously, or the order in which they were shown sequentially. All this information should be made available to the defence*. This rule and the following aim at making it possible to check the quality of a line up afterwards. If the outcome of the procedure is that

the suspect is identified, the defence may be eager to check the quality of the procedure. This is obviously only possible if all relevant information is documented and retained. Wagenaar (1989) distinguishes simultaneous and sequential line ups. By now, there is some evidence indicating that sequential line ups may be superior to simultaneous ones in terms of diagnostic value. For example, in the previously mentioned meta-analysis by Clark et al. (2008), the accuracy rates of witnesses in 81 simultaneous and 9 sequential line ups were compared. In the former condition, the true positive likelihood was 47% and the false positive likelihood was 14%, yielding a likelihood ratio (after weighting) of 5.5. In the sequential line ups, performance was slightly better with 40% true positives and only 8% false positives, yielding a weighted likelihood ratio of 6.4. In another meta-analysis, Steblay et al. (2011) cumulated findings of 49 studies on simultaneous and sequential line ups. These authors reported an average likelihood ratio of 5.8 for positive identifications in simultaneous, and 7.7 for sequential line ups. They also reported likelihood ratios for nonidentifications and came to 1.9 for the simultaneous and 2.9 for the sequential line up. Notably, the stronger diagnosticity of sequential line ups may be due to the circumstance that the witness is prevented from picking the individual who matches his recollection of the culprit best. Hence, in the sequential line up, it is impossible to compare individuals and choose relatively, by comparison. For each shown individual, a dichotomous, absolute judgement must be made, before the next one is shown. To achieve these circumstances, a few additional rules must be followed. For example, it should be forbidden that the witness returns to a previously shown individual. Once an individual is rejected, the sequential line up moves on, and one cannot go back. Further, the witness should not be instructed how many individuals will be shown, in order to prevent that he will identify the last, merely because the witness knows that he is the last. It is also custom that the suspect should not be presented in the first position, to exclude the possibility that he is identified by a witness who does not fully understand the procedure and simply identifies the first individual.

35. *Live line ups* (i.e., *in person) should be documented with photographs, These pictures should be made available to the defence*. The rationale behind rule 35 is identical to rule 34.
36. *Names and contact information of foils should be retained, but not automatically be made available to the defence*. Foils may be able to give valuable information that sheds light on the validity of the line up identification. Thus, in order to check the procedure in hindsight, it may come in handy to be able to contact the foils.
37. *If possible, live line ups should be documented audiovisually*. Again, this rule rests on the same idea as does rule number 35 and others.
38. *Foils and suspect need to be instructed properly on how they should behave in order to prevent leaking cues to the witness during the procedure*. This rule seeks to avoid bias caused (unconsciously) by the behaviour of the individuals in the line up. Imagine that the suspect is depressed and/or is sleep deprived, and that these circumstances leak from his posture, whereas all foils feel fine.

Similar unfairness may be the result of walking speed, looking around (or not), and displaying facial emotion. One would hope that such bias causing the suspect to somehow stand out can be avoided by instruction.

39. *Recent alterations in the appearance of the suspect should be made undone as much as possible.* Imagine that a witness describes a perpetrator who wore a moustache. The suspect, however, does not have a moustache and informs the police that he used to have a moustache but recently shaved it off. In this case, the disappearance of the moustache may hinder the identification of the suspect (if he is the perpetrator). It is then recommendable to have the suspect (and all foils) regrow a moustache, in order to make it match the description of the perpetrator. Obviously, the undoing of alterations only pertains to changes that occurred after the crime, yet before the identification procedure.
40. *If possible, the police officer supervising the identification procedure should be unaware who is the suspect.* This rule prevents the supervising police officer from (subconsciously) sending cues to the witness to steer him to identify the suspect. The police may influence the witness in numerous ways, ranging from remarks such as 'Are you sure you do not recognise anyone …take another look at number 2' to coughing when the witness is looking at the suspect, or even by looking oneself at the suspect disproportionally long. Wells and Luus (1990) argue that the line up can be approached as a scientific experiment, in which the experiment leader (cf. the supervising police officer) should be blind to the condition to which the participant is allocated. Thus, they think of 'line ups as experiments'. Taking this approach makes it also completely logical that there should be foils, who can be said to fulfil the role of controls needed to exclude alternative explanations for a positive outcome, if any.
41. *The exposure time to the photos or persons should be limited to a few minutes.* There is some evidence suggesting that valid identifications tend to be made quite rapidly, even within seconds. Dunning and Perretta (2002) proposed that in a simultaneous line up consisting of five to six pictures, a neat cut-off would be 10–12 s. Participants who decided within this time were accurate in 90% of the cases. Participants who needed longer were only 50% accurate. This suggests that exposure time should indeed be short.
42. *It is important that all relevant details in the preparation and during the exposure* (e.g., *remarks by the witness) are documented in the report.* This rule is another failsafe to enable interested parties in checking the quality of the identification procedure afterwards.
43. *The witness should not receive feedback on his identification.* Withholding feedback from the witness on his performance serves several purposes. First, it prevents the witness from giving away the line up to other witnesses, if any. That is, it prevents the witness from making remarks such as 'I just completed the identification procedure and identified number 2, the police officer thanked me and said that I picked the suspect'. Second, it is recommendable to obtain a confidence statement from the witness, if there is a positive identification (see rule number 47). However, confidence can be steered enormously by feedback. Particularly, if the witness is informed that he picked the right one, confidence

will unduly inflate. Luus and Wells (1994) carried out a classic experiment illustrating the effect of feedback on confidence. They made 140 undergraduates, in couples, witness to a theft. Participants were invited to participate in a study on their capacity to match voices to faces. Hence, their picture was taken to be used as stimulus materials for later participants. When they entered the room where the study was to take place, they saw a woman taking a piece of equipment and leaving the room through another door. Once the experiment leader followed participants into the room, he allegedly noticed that a crucial piece of lab equipment was missing, and concluded that this must have been stolen by the individual who just left the room. He also expressed suspicion that the thief was likely to be a former participant, because no one else knew that there was valuable equipment in the room. Luckily, pictures of all six female participants so far had been taken. The experiment leader asked the participants to look at the six pictures to see if they could recognise any of them as the thief. Each participant was taken to a different room to undergo the line up. Once the participant had made an identification, the experiment leader would in some instances give feedback. Sometimes he left the room, allegedly to go to the other participants, and came back in two minutes with updated feedback. Ultimately, a police officer (actually a stooge) asked the participants how confident they were about their identification on a scale from 1 through 10. Unknown to participants, the theft was actually staged, and the sole purpose of the study was to test the effect of feedback on confidence. There were nine feedback conditions: (1) control condition without feedback, (2) the other witness identified the same photo, (3) the other witness identified another photo, (4) the other witness rejected the line up, (5) the other witness identified another photo that was actually implausible (the picture was quite different from the thief), (6) the initial feedback was that the other witness identified another photo, but when returning two minutes later, the experiment leader said that he had made a mistake and that the other witness had actually identified the same photo (different-same), (7) feedback mirrored to condition 6, that is, initial positive feedback, followed by corrected negative feedback (same-different), (8) initial positive feedback, followed by the comment that the experiment leader actually was unsure what the other witness had said (same-withdraw), and (9) different-withdraw.

For research purpose, the authors wanted all participants to make a false positive identification. They had four instruments to achieve this: (1) the thief was not in the line up, so any identification was by definition false, (2) five pictures were quite different from the thief, whereas one resembled her, (3) participants were not informed that they were allowed to reject the line up, and (4) the exposure time during the theft was short. All in all, 136 witnesses made a false positive identification (97%). Their confidence ratings are displayed in Fig. 3.1. The interview in which participants rated their confidence in their identification was video-recorded and later shown to a new sample of 378 undergraduates. These observers were asked to rate

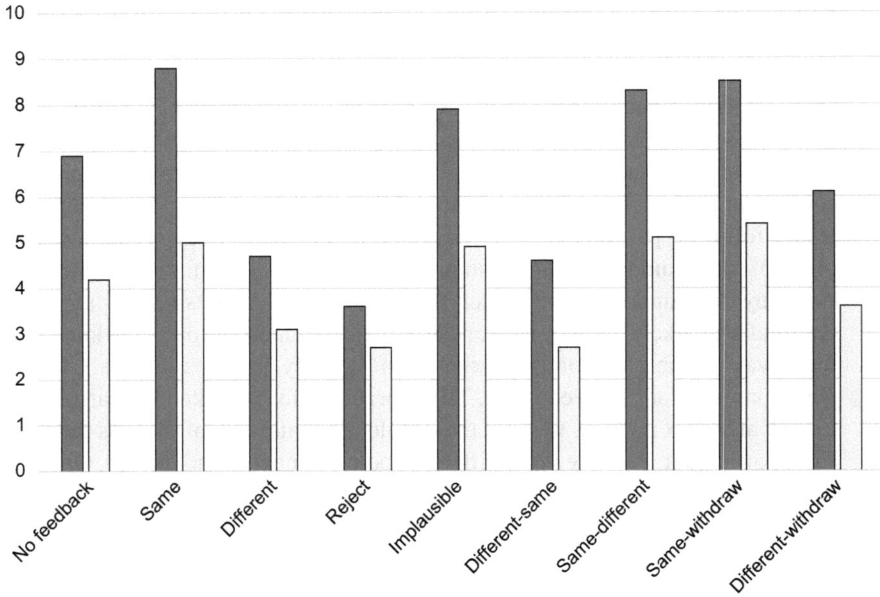

Fig. 3.1 Confidence (1–10, grey) and perceived accuracy (1–7, white) ratings. (Luus & Wells, 1994)

their estimate of how accurate the identification made by the witness was, on a scale from 1 through 7. These ratings are also included in Fig. 3.1.

As can be seen, the effect of feedback was considerable, with positive feedback resulting in increased confidence, and negative feedback resulting in decreased confidence. Note that the feedback that the other witness identified an implausible picture was perceived as positive feedback. Note further that there was a strong primacy effect in the latter four conditions: The initial feedback, not the corrected feedback, steered confidence. Finally, the data neatly illustrate that the observers used the self-reported confidence of the witnesses as the main factor to build their estimation of the accuracy upon (see also Hasel & Kassin, 2009, for similar findings on the detrimental effect of feedback on confidence).

44. *The defence lawyer should be admitted to the line up procedure. If the suspect's lawyer is present, he can check whether the police comply with the crucial rules for the proper conduction of the identification procedure. Thus, this rule is another safeguard making it possible to check the procedure. In addition, the police, knowing that the defence is watching, may do their best even more to optimise the procedure.*
45. *If the witness merely reports a resemblance between a person in the line up and the perpetrator, this does not count as an identification.* It is important that the witness actively positively identifies the suspect, if it is to be considered evidence against the suspect. A mere resemblance does not suffice as an identification. Admittedly, the suspect may well resemble the perpetrator yet not be him.

46. *An identification that follows a long (*i.e., *more than a few minutes) period of deliberation does not count as an identification.* This rule is a mirrored and stronger version of rule number 41. The idea is that accurate identifications occur rapidly upon seeing the individuals in the line up. Long deliberations are not needed. Moreover, longer periods of deliberation are associated with inaccuracy of the identification (Dunning & Perretta, 2002).
47. *If the witness reports uncertainties, these should be documented in the report.* Wagenaar (1989) argued that expressed uncertainty may reflect inaccuracy of the outcome. In his line of reasoning, self-reported confidence should be high as a prerequisite, whereas reported uncertainties suppress the evidentiary strength of the identification. In a meta-analysis of the relation between confidence and accuracy, Sporer et al. (1995) found a positive correlation ($r = .37$) between confidence and accuracy for witnesses who make a positive identification, but no significant correlation ($r = .12$) for the non-choosers. In an alternative analysis, they concluded that witnesses who made a correct positive identification rated their confidence on average at about 76%, whereas mistaken witnesses got stuck at 54%. For the non-choosers, witnesses who correctly rejected the line up rated their confidence at 71%, while the incorrect rejecters got stuck at 64%. Interestingly, in recent literature, self-reported confidence is argued to be a sign of accuracy (Wixted & Wells, 2017). Note that considering uncertainty to indicate inaccuracy is not necessarily the same as considering confidence to support accuracy. This is especially important in a criminal context that is guided by the principle of the presumption of innocence. In such a context, it may well be considered dubious to place more trust in a piece of incriminating evidence merely because the witness is confident. Notwithstanding, Wells et al. (2020) argue that 'eyewitness confidence is a useful cue to the accuracy of a witness's decision' (p. 22). They recommend that self-reported confidence in an identification be registered on a scale from 0% through 100%. They add that this rating should be elicited immediately after the identification: 'Note that forcing the witnesses to withhold their confidence reports for as little as 5 min has been found to undermine the predictive value of confidence' (p. 22).
48. *An identification in court is not evidence of identity.* It may happen in a court session that a witness is asked by the district's attorney whether he can identify the perpetrator, and that the witness responds that he recognises the suspect. Whereas this may leave a strong impression, it does actually not suffice as an evidence-worthy identification. Firstly, this identification actually boils down to a show up, which does, according to Wagenaar (1989), by definition not suffice as evidence. Further, even if an identification in a show up is taken as evidence, the circumstances in court are not optimal. For example, it is obvious to the witness who the suspect is. This may introduce a bias, or even experienced commitment towards a positive identification when invited. Also, the exposure time of the witness to the suspect is far too long, considering that the witness remains on the witness stand for some time.
49. *If a rule of proper line up procedure is violated without documentation or explanation in the report, this should result in inadmissibility of the identification.*

This rule seeks to pressure the police into conducting a proper identification procedure, including a complete and accurate report of the procedure. Small, probably harmless deviations from the rules and guidelines should be documented. Failure to do so should meet a severe penalty, namely that the incriminating evidentiary power of the identification is reduced to zero.

50. *If a violation of a rule of proper line up procedure is concluded to suppress the validity of the identification, the identification should be declared inadmissible, even if the violation is documented and explained in the report.* Some of Wagenaar's (1989) rules are more important than others. For example, if rule number 44 is violated and the defence attorney is not present during the identification procedure, this does not necessarily undo all the evidentiary power of the identification. By contrast, if it turns out that the line up was biased (a violation of rule number 32), this does destroy the surplus value of the line up compared to a show up. Even worse: The suspect might have been better off in a show up than in a biased line up because the latter literally points the witness in de direction of the suspect.

Controlling all system variables as prescribed by Wagenaar's (1989) 50 rules cannot guarantee that a positive identification is true. Obviously, scientific research cannot yield accuracy rates for all possible circumstances (particularly estimator variables) surrounding eyewitness identification evidence in any particular case. Generally, if no other information is available, it seems fair to say that the average evidentiary power of a positive identification in a line up procedure, expressed in a likelihood ratio is about 5 through 8 (Clark et al., 2008; Steblay et al., 2011), and about 2 in a show up (Steblay et al., 2003). Quite generally, the exonerating strength of nonidentifications is about 2–3 in a line up procedure, and slightly less than 2 in a show up (Steblay et al., 2003, 2011).

Finally, it should be noted that the rules and guidelines discussed in this paragraph are not legal rules. They are the result of psychological research. It is up to the legal decision maker to decide whether or not he wishes to apply the rules. Indeed, judges and juries may not even be fully familiar with these rules. Moreover, the rules are not even generally accepted among psychological experts. By now, various studies in various countries have shown that there is some disagreement between experts (Benton et al., 2006; Kassin et al., 1989, 2001) and professional judges (Magnussen et al., 2008; Wise & Safer, 2004).

3.2 The Identification Evidence in This Case

In my view, most of Wagenaar's (1989) recommendations for setting up a good line up had been met in this instance. However, there were some circumstances that did suppress the strength of the identification of the suspect. In my report, I noted that the woman had seen the suspect before the robbery, at least in his account. This introduced the risk that she might identify him because she recognised him from this earlier encounter. However, she did not identify him at all, so this problem did not occur. Meanwhile, the possibility that suspect and witness had met before did not stop the police from conducting a line up. This risk of a false fame effect might be present for the identification by the son. It was not documented whether the son had been present during the alleged visit by the suspect as a salesman, but he did testify that he had seen the suspect between the robbery and the line up procedure. If the son was mistaken at that time (i.e., he saw the suspect in the street, and thought he recognised him, whereas in fact the suspect was not the perpetrator), his recollection of the perpetrator may have been overwritten by that of the suspect, potentially causing a false identification later on. Hence, the repeated encounter with the suspect hindered the assumption that if the witness identified the suspect, this can have absolutely only one reason, namely their encounter during the crime. For a truly strong identification, the witness must have seen the perpetrator (= suspect) only once, that is, during the crime.

Strikingly, Wells et al. (2020) argue against this position, when they say that if the witness new the perpetrator beforehand, this increases identification accuracy: 'prior familiarity with the culprit ... generally increases the accuracy of a witness's description and identification' (p. 10). Whereas this is true, Wagenaar (1989) would subsequently advise against a line up. Obviously, if the police take the trouble of setting up a line up, it is still to be determined whether the suspect is the perpetrator, and thus, alleged familiarity between the witness and the suspect cannot by definition be taken as familiarity between the witness and the culprit. De Jong et al. (2005) went so far as to say that whereas line ups are recommendable if the witness saw an unfamiliar culprit, 'identification problems of a different kind may occur with persons already known to a witness ... (e.g., nephew) ... a subsequent identity test in which you are asked to identify your nephew is of course useless and even nonsensical' (p. 88).

A second point was that the woman did not identify the suspect. If some evidential value is attributed to the identification by the son, would it then be fair to subtract some because of the mother's nonidentification? If we attribute a likelihood ratio of 7.7 to the identification by the son (not considering the possibility of a false fame effect due to repeated exposure), then a likelihood ratio of (1: 2.9 =) 0.34 for the negative evidence is also in line (Steblay et al., 2011), yielding a combined evidentiary power of 2.62. In sum, I recommended that the identification had limited power, particularly in combination with the nonidentification by the woman.

The appeal court was not convinced by the evidence. In reference to my report, they considered the identification to be weak evidence. Further, they could not refute the suspect's alternative account of how his cigarette got at the crime scene. Finally, they attributed exonerating value to the suspect's alibi, which was corroborated by his friend.

References

Benton, T. R., Ross, D. F., Bradshaw, E., Thomas, W. N., & Bradshaw, G. S. (2006). Eyewitness memory is still not common sense: Comparing jurors, judges and law enforcement to eyewitness experts. *Applied Cognitive Psychology, 20*, 115–129.

Carmichael, L. C., Hogan, H. P., & Walter, A. A. (1932). An experimental study of the effect of language on the reproduction of visually perceived forms. *Journal of Experimental Psychology, 15*, 73–86.

Clark, S. E., & Wells, G. L. (2008). On the diagnosticity of multiple-witness identifications. *Law and Human Behavior, 32*, 406–422.

Clark, S. E., Howell, R. T., & Davey, S. L. (2008). Regularities in eyewitness identification. *Law and Human Behavior, 32*, 187–218.

De Jong, M., Wagenaar, W. A., Wolters, G., & Verstijnen, I. M. (2005). Familiar face recognition as a function of distance and illumination: A practical tool for use in the courtroom. *Psychology, Crime & Law, 11*, 87–97.

Doob, A. N., & Kirshenbaum, H. M. (1973). Bias in police lineups: Partial remembering. *Journal of Police Science and Administration, 1*, 287–293.

Dunning, D., & Perretta, S. (2002). Automaticity and eyewitness accuracy: A 10-to-12-seconds rule for distinguishing accurate from inaccurate positive identifications. *Journal of Applied Psychology, 87*, 951–962.

Hasel, L. E., & Kassin, S. M. (2009). On the presumption of evidentiary independence: Can confessions corrupt eyewitness identifications? *Psychological Science, 20*, 122–126.

Jacoby, L. L., Kelley, C. M., Brown, J., & Jasechko, J. (1989). Becoming famous overnight: Limits on the ability to avoid unconscious influences of the past. *Journal of Personality and Social Psychology, 56*, 326–338.

Kassin, S. M., Ellsworth, P. C., & Smith, V. L. (1989). The "general acceptance" of psychological research on eyewitness testimony: A survey of the experts. *American Psychologist, 44*, 1089–1098.

Kassin, S. M., Tubb, V. A., Hosch, H. M., & Memon, A. (2001). On the "general acceptance" of eyewitness testimony research. *American Psychologist, 56*, 405–416.

Loftus, E. F. (1976). Unconscious transference in eyewitness identification. *Law and Psychology Review, 2*, 93–98.

Luus, C. A. E., & Wells, G. L. (1994). The malleability of eyewitness confidence. Co-witness and perseverance effects. *Journal of Applied Psychology, 79*, 714–723.

Magnussen, S., Wise, R. A., Raja, A. Q., Safer, M. A., Pawlenko, N., & Stridbeck, U. (2008). What judges know about eyewitness testimony: A comparison of Norwegian and US judges. *Psychology, Crime & Law, 14*, 177–188.

Meissner, C. A., & Brigham, J. C. (2001). A meta-analysis of the verbal overshadowing effect in face identification. *Applied Cognitive Psychology, 15*, 603–616.

Rassin, E. (2013). Presence bias and the insensitivity to the diagnosticity of nonidentifications. *Psychology, Crime & Law, 19*, 203–214.

Sporer, S. L., Penrod, S. D., Read, J. D., & Cutler, B. L. (1995). Choosing, confidence, and accuracy: A meta-analysis of the confidence-accuracy relation in eyewitness identification studies. *Psychological Bulletin, 118*, 315–327.

Steblay, N., Dysart, J., Fulero, S., & Lindsay, R. C. L. (2003). Eyewitness accuracy rates in police showup and lineup presentations: A meta-analytic comparison. *Law and Human Behavior, 27*, 523–540.

Steblay, N. K., Dysart, J. E., & Wells, G. L. (2011). Seventy-two tests of the sequential lineup superiority effect: A meta-analysis and policy discussion. *Psychology, Public Policy, and Law, 17*, 99–139.

Tredoux, C. (1998). Statistical inference on measures of lineup fairness. *Law and Human Behavior, 22*, 217–237.

Wagenaar, W. A. (1989). *Identifying Ivan: A case study in legal psychology*. University Press.

Wells, G. L., & Lindsay, R. C. L. (1980). On estimating the diagnosticity of eyewitness nonidentifications. *Psychological Bulletin, 88*, 776–784.
Wells, G. L., & Luus, E. (1990). Police lineups as experiments: Social methodology as a framework for properly-conducted lineups. *Personality and Social Psychology Bulletin, 16*, 106–117.
Wells, G. L., & Olson, E. A. (2002). Eyewitness identification: Information gain from incriminating and exonerating behaviours. *Journal of Experimental Psychology: Applied, 8*, 155–167.
Wells, G. L., Bull Kovera, M., Douglass, A. B., Brewer, N., Meissner, C. A., & Wixted, J. T. (2020). Policy and procedure recommendations for the collection and preservation of eyewitness identification evidence. *Law and Human Behavior, 44*, 3–36.
Wise, R. A., & Safer, M. A. (2004). What US judges know and believe about eyewitness testimony. *Applied Cognitive Psychology, 18*, 427–443.
Wixted, J. T., & Wells, G. L. (2017). The relationship between eyewitness confidence and identification accuracy: A new synthesis. *Psychological Science in the Public Interest, 18*, 10–65.

Chapter 4
Popeye and an Obscure Mix of Identification Procedures

Late one evening in December 2012, three men were walking in the street in Amsterdam when they saw a car (Audi RS4) approaching rapidly. Through an open car window, they were shot at. Two men were killed. The third one ran away, and was followed and chased by several assailants who had gotten out of the car. Eventually, the third victim got away by jumping into the canal. Because the victim ran various blocks, while being shot at repeatedly, there were many witnesses who saw part of the incident from their apartment window. In fact, some people called the alarm number while the assassination attack was still ongoing. Witnesses informed the police by phone in which direction they had seen the Audi leave the crime scene. With this information, the police had two motor colleagues wait at a certain intersection where they expected the Audi to drive by soon. It so happened, but the perpetrators did not stop. By contrast, they drove on rapidly through the improvised barricade, and opened fire at the police. The police returned fire, and during this exchange, the police shot a windshield. Nonetheless, the Audi got away. It is found abandoned soon after. Nearby, the perpetrators apparently threw away several firearms and ammunition into the water. The third victim was unharmed, and was interviewed by the police. He claimed to have seen who pointed the gun and shot at him. He knew this person and spontaneously mentioned the nickname of the man, Popeye, who henceforth became the suspect.

Popeye's defence attorney asked for a (psychological) opinion on the strength of the identification evidence against his client. He also informed me that Popeye's DNA was found in the passenger's seat of the Audi. However, they were planning an activity-level defence, saying that Popeye admitted having been in the car, but not at the time of the shooting. It turned out that Popeye and the victim were part of rivalling criminal gangs. According to the lawyer, it was not uncommon for them to steal a car, use it for several days, and then abandon it somewhere.

ECLI:NL:GHAMS:2020:915

E. Rassin, *Case Studies in Legal Psychology*,
https://doi.org/10.1007/978-3-031-44931-4_4

Obviously, the strength of the identification is modulated by several factors. Note that the identification in this case took place in the street. It was during the assassination attempt that the victim thought to see Popeye. All relevant factors are hence estimator variables. Think of the distance from which the victim saw the shooter, the illumination, emotional state of the victim, expectancy effects, and the exposure time. All these factors may have affected the victim's perception and recollection of the event. To estimate the strength of the eyewitness identification, I referred to a study by de Jong et al. (2005) in which the effect of distance and illumination on recognition of a familiar face was tested. From the case file, it could be derived that the illumination at the time of the incident was around 5 lux (moderately illuminated city street at night), and the smallest distance between the witness and the perpetrator was at least 5 meters.

De Jong et al. (2005) presented pictures of public figures (e.g., actors and politicians) to 65 undergraduates at various distances and levels of illumination. They registered the likelihood of a true positive identification (i.e., the identification of the public figure), but also the likelihood of a false positive identification (i.e., the likelihood that the participant recognises the public figure whereas in fact the person in the photograph is not the public figure but a lookalike sharing the same description). The true and false positive likelihoods as a function of distance and illumination are presented in Table 4.1.

As can be seen, illumination and distance seem to affect identification accuracy in the expected direction. Based on these findings, the authors (re)introduced their rule of thumb, known as the rule of 15: For a valid identification with a likelihood ratio of at least 15, the identification should take place at no more than 15 m, and under no less than 15 lux.

Table 4.1 True (bold) and false positive likelihoods (De Jong et al., 2005)

Distance (metres)	Illumination level (lux)								
	0.3	2	3	5	10	30	150	300	3000
3	**0**	**79**	**100**	**100**	**93**	**96**	**94**	**97**	**97**
	0	0	5	0	8	3	0	0	0
5	**0**	**68**	**89**	**94**	**94**	**97**	**92**	**92**	**100**
	0	14	8	14	3	6	0	7	3
7		**63**	**63**	**89**	**93**	**93**	**97**	**96**	**90**
		3	10	3	6	3	6	3	0
12			**60**	**70**	**76**	**81**	**80**	**92**	**100**
			3	6	6	5	3	5	2
20				**32**	**52**	**65**	**77**	**79**	**100**
				6	14	9	13	6	14
30					**20**	**29**	**32**	**45**	**40**
					10	8	11	8	5
40						**7**	**17**	**17**	**30**
						3	5	10	2

Given a 5 m distance and 5 lux illumination, there is a likelihood of 94% of recognizing someone we know. Under these conditions, there is a likelihood of 14% to (mis)recognize someone who is, in fact, somebody else merely resembling our acquaintance. These two likelihoods can be used to calculate the likelihood ratio, which is (94%: 14% =) 6.7. Hence, I wrote in my report: 'The likelihood ratio of the identification, given the perceptual circumstances, is approximately 6.7 (…). However, there were additional circumstances that threaten the validity of the identification, that are not included in the estimation of this likelihood ratio, such as time pressure, stress, and movement of the perpetrator (…). Therefore, the precise likelihood ratio may well be smaller than 6.7 (…). It is impossible to give a more precise estimate'.

Soon after I had sent my report to the lawyer, and he had presented it to the prosecution, the lawyer showed me a written reaction by the district's attorney: 'The expert's computation is based on the case information provided by the defence. Some information, supporting the identification, was lacking. For example, the expert was not informed about the important forensic finding that the suspect's DNA was secured on the headrest of the Audi. In our view, a correct computation of the likelihood ratio of the identification should have considered this important finding. Hence, by supplying the expert with limited information, the defence affected the computation. We cannot know to what likelihood ratio the expert would have concluded, had he been given information about the DNA evidence. Conclusion: the report has very limited value since it was based on incomplete case information'.

Obviously, the likelihood ratio of eyewitness identification is not affected by the presence of other evidence. Only when deciding on the guilt of the defendant, the judge will have to consider all the evidence conjointly. The district's attorney's argument would have probably more easily been recognizable as irrelevant, had he reversely argued that the DNA evidence should be considered to be stronger than the DNA expert had presented, merely because an eyewitness also identified the suspect. Of course, the strength of a DNA finding is not affected by whether or not the suspect was identified by an eyewitness, nor by any other evidence. Logically, this also works the other way around.

In 2020, the Court of appeal handled this case. By then, more information had been uncovered. Popeye had changed lawyers. My report was not part of the case file. The court argued as follows. First, as to the identification of the suspect by the victim, it became clear to me that this had been more problematic than initially revealed to me. The victim had claimed that he recognized Popeye as one of the shooters. However, the suspect had six brothers and many of them if not all were known as Popeye. The victim had also claimed that Popeye was the oldest brother, whereas the suspect was in fact the second. Three months after the assault, the police showed photos of various brothers to the victim who then pointed out the suspect. This identification procedure is difficult to interpret. It is not a good evidential line up, because if for no other reason, all persons shown were potential suspects. Guidelines by Wagenaar (1989) would argue against conducting a line up in this instance, because the victim knew Popeye beforehand (note that Wells et al., 2020, would see this as a reason to set up an evidence line up). Popeye's new defence lawyers criticized the identification because it was not a proper line up. They also argued that the suspect was wearing a blue prison suit as opposed to the other brothers. This will bias the identification. The prosecution argued that a mugshot series is only in place if there is no suspect yet. Hence, the current procedure was a mix, and definitely not a line up. The court decided that regulations and guidelines regarding eyewitness identification procedures only pertain to confrontations in person (live). And because in this case, photos were used, it is out of place to criticize the quality of the procedure. In sum, the victim's statement that it was Popeye, including the identification in the identification procedure, was admissible as evidence.

Second, as to the suspect's DNA on the headrest of the Audi, technical analysis yielded the conclusion that the DNA found was 1 billion times more likely if it was from the suspect than if it were from a random other person. But then, the defence argued that the alternative hypothesis in this case is not that the DNA was from a random third person, but from another Popeye brother. Reanalysis of the data yielded a likelihood of 60,000 in favour of the primary hypothesis.

A third piece of evidence was a piece of glass found in a shoe. It had turned out that the suspect's wife owned a piece of land quite nearby where the Audi was found. On this land, there was a shed. In there, the police found sports shoes that allegedly belonged to the suspect. These shoes were analysed, and turned out to contain 35 small pieces of fractured glass. These glass pieces were compared (as to structure and breaking index) with the shattered car window. Of 33 fragments it was concluded that they did not belong to the car window. Of one piece it was said to provide moderately strong support for the primary hypothesis (i.e., likelihood ratio between 100 and 10,000). One other piece was concluded to provide weak support (likelihood ratio between 2 and 10). This finding fits in the hypothesis that the suspect ran to this shed after abandoning the car, and changed clothes there. Hence, the sports shoes were worn during the assault. The defence resisted this evidence, because according to them, the glass used as comparison was drawn from just 17 sources, none of which were Audi shields. The court used the glass as evidence nonetheless.

Fourth, DNA was found on the ammunition that was thrown into the water. A DNA sample found on a shell of a Colt was examined and concluded to be 80,000 times more likely if it was from the suspect than if it were from an unknown random other person. Obviously, this finding too fits well with the hypothesis that the suspect was one of the perpetrators.

Finally, the court noted that the suspect brought forward an alibi for the assault. But he did so not before April 2013 (i.e., 4 months after the crime). He claimed to have been in a bar. However, when asked, none of the regular customers or personnel could confirm this alibi. This last findings was not construed as evidence against the suspect, but it was mentioned in the deliberations.

In sum, the eyewitness identification, the DNA on the Audi's headrest, the glass fragments in the shoe, and the DNA on the bullet convinced the court that the suspect was indeed one of the assailants. Given the severity of the crime (primarily double murder and attempted murder), and the 18-page-long prior sheet, the court convicted the suspect to lifelong imprisonment. As is done mostly, the court merely summed up the pieces of evidence used to reach conviction. However, given that most of the evidence in this case was technical in nature and evaluated in terms of likelihood ratios, the case lends itself perfectly to demonstrate what a Bayesian approach would look like. Let us say that the initial testimony of the surviving witness serves as prior odds. Given that the nickname Popeye reasonably applied to seven people, the prior odds are arguably (14%: 86% =) 0.16. The two glass fragments had a lower bound value of 100 and 2. The two DNA traces had likelihood ratios of 60,000 and 80,000. All this results in posterior odds of 153,600,000,000. The corresponding likelihood that the suspect was one of the perpetrators is then 99.9999999993%. Obviously, this Bayesian analysis points in the same direction as the narrative approach taken by the court.

References

De Jong, M., Wagenaar, W. A., Wolters, G., & Verstijnen, I. M. (2005). Familiar face recognition as a function of distance and illumination: A practical tool for use in the courtroom. *Psychology, Crime & Law, 11*, 87–97.

Wagenaar, W. A. (1989). *Identifying Ivan: A case study in legal psychology*. University Press.

Wells, G. L., Bull Kovera, M., Douglass, A. B., Brewer, N., Meissner, C. A., & Wixted, J. T. (2020). Policy and procedure recommendations for the collection and preservation of eyewitness identification evidence. *Law and Human Behavior, 44*, 3–36.

Chapter 5
Delayed Allegation of Sexual Assault, Repression and Psychotherapy

Somewhere in 2015, two female friends in their early 13, file allegation of sexual abuse against the male owner of a cafeteria. Over 15 years ago, the two friends were regular babysitters for the suspect and his wife. While they would go out to work in their establishment, one of the girls (then about 15 years of age) would babysit the two children. Sometimes, the suspect would come home before his wife did, and in these moments, he would abuse the babysitter. The reason for the delay in allegation is that the two friends had only recently become aware of the abuse. Until then, the recollection of the abuse had been repressed. Nonetheless, they did not feel completely happy, and sought psychotherapeutic help. One underwent hypnotherapy, in the hope of finding out why she felt so miserable. The other took group sessions of unknown composition and purpose. During these therapies, they recovered the memories of the abuse. They then took Eye Movement Desensitisation and Reprocessing (EMDR) to get over the newly recovered traumatic memory. Meanwhile, they frequently talked to each other about the abuse, and tried to convince a third friend that she had also been abused by the suspect, though this woman was not convinced and did not press charges. The two women once went to the suspect's home, to refresh their memory of the crimes. At some point, their therapists encouraged them to file allegation. The suspect denied. He testified that he did not even know the two women. In fact, there was no information to corroborate that the women had ever babysitted for the suspect.

5.1 Criteria-Based Content Analysis (CBCA)

A psychological expert witness, Dr. Wolters, had already given opinion about the reliability of the allegations. Based on a technique akin to CBCA he came to the conclusion that they were reliable. However, the court did not completely trust the

---

ECLI:NL:RBDHA:2018:13856

E. Rassin, *Case Studies in Legal Psychology*,
https://doi.org/10.1007/978-3-031-44931-4_5

work of the expert, because at the time of his analysis, the casefile was not yet complete. Therefore, the court decided that a second opinion was needed. This initiative came primarily from the defence because the prosecution was in fact satisfied with the positive conclusion of the initial expert.

CBCA has dominated the literature on verbal lie detection for some decades now. In the words of Oberlader et al. (2016, p. 441): CBCA 'is probably the most widely used veracity assessment technique in the world'. In essence, CBCA is a list of 19 criteria with which a literally transcribed testimony can be scrutinised. The criteria are framed in the direction of credibility, that is, if a particular criterion is met by the testimony, this is considered to support the veracity of the testimony. The criteria are as follows.

1. The testimony should have a logical structure. That is, the content should not be bizarre.
2. The testimony is an unstructured reproduction of the event. That is, the narrative is reproduced spontaneously, and therefore not too slick, smooth. For example, there are time jumps and spontaneous self-corrections.
3. The testimony is rich in details (excluding repetitions).
4. The event is contextually embedded. The witness places the event in time and place.
5. The narrative includes three-stage interactions (e.g., comment, reply, and reply).
6. The narrative includes verbal quotes.
7. Unexpected complications that happened during the event are mentioned. For example, the witness reports that an unknowing third party walked by during the incident.
8. The testimony includes unusual, but realistic and in the context meaningful details.
9. There are some seemingly superfluous details in the narrative.
10. The witness reports details that he apparently does not understand, but describes correctly nonetheless. For example, a child may report a conversation between two adults, and while the child does not understand the content of that conversation, it is clear that the content, as reproduced by the child witness, has a logical structure.
11. The testimony includes reference to external yet related events. For example, a child witness in a sex crime case may report that the suspect had previously made sexual remarks in other situations.
12. The witness reports on his subjective experiences (e.g., feelings and thoughts).
13. The witness reports on estimated subjective experiences of the perpetrator (e.g., feelings and thoughts; overt behaviours are excluded from this criterion).
14. The witness makes spontaneous corrections to his statement.
15. The witness spontaneously makes remarks about memory failure. This is to be distinguished from replying 'I don't know' when asked for specific details.
16. The witness spontaneously reports that part of the statement may appear incredible.

17. The testimony includes some self-blaming or self-depreciation (e.g., including that the event was partly due to himself).
18. The witness pardons the perpetrator, minimises the severity, or does not jump at the opportunity to blame the perpetrator.
19. Inclusion of details that are unique for the alleged crime (e.g., in case of sexual assault, when the witness describes in detail certain body parts of the perpetrator, such as birth marks).

It is important to appreciate that the 19 CBCA criteria differ in nature, and in various ways. To understand this, the development of CBCA must be considered. It goes back to a notion forwarded by Undeutsch (1967). The so-called Undeutsch hypothesis states, first of all, that children can give valid testimony (which was at that time a novel insight), and moreover, that it is possible to detect truth and falsity in children's testimonies. This discrimination leans one two ideas, namely (1) that truth tellers are more spontaneous, and hence, less concentrated on impression management than liars, and (2) that children are unable to produce certain details when fabricating a narrative (Steller & Köhnken, 1989). Hence, after a couple of generic criteria (1–3), CBCA contains motivational criteria (e.g., numbers 14–18) and cognitive criteria (e.g., numbers 4–13). Indeed, CBCA was originally meant to be used for the validation of children's testimonies. Obviously, older children and adults can be expected to evade detection with CBCA criteria, because they are better at lying than are young children. Note that CBCA was not only exclusively meant to be applied to children's testimonies, but also particularly in sexual abuse cases. Consequently, some criteria are simply not applicable in all cases. Thus, while presence of criteria is considered to support credibility, their absence is not considered to indicate falsity (Ruby & Brigham, 1997).

CBCA is a part of statement validity analysis (SVA), which also includes a validity checklist (VC). The psychologist who evaluates the validity of a statement not only completes the CBCA but also the VC. The VC consists of the following topics that fall outside of the testimony at hand.

1. Possible cognitive and emotional limitations.
2. Appropriate language and knowledge displayed by the witness.
3. Appropriateness of emotions displayed during the interview.
4. Suggestibility.
5. The quality of interview procedures, such as rapport building, instructions, and free recall elicitation. Ideally, the police conduct a special SVA interview which is characterised by the absence of closed and leading questions, so that there is only a free recall.
6. Possible influence of the interviewer on the content of the testimony (e.g., leading questions, coercion, or other suggestive interventions).
7. Possible motives to give a false testimony.
8. Possible suspicious disclosure circumstances, or major inconsistencies over time.
9. Possible third-party influences on the witness (e.g., suggestion or coercion).
10. Lack of realism.

11. Inconsistency in core aspects of the testified event.
12. Contradictory evidence.
13. Conflict with general knowledge of similar crimes.

Note that the criteria in the VC are, unlike those in CBCA, sometimes framed in the direction of falsity. This is one of the reasons why the VC is a crucial counterpart of CBCA within the SVA. Notably, and unfortunately, however, CBCA is oftentimes used in practice in absence of the VC, possibly because it is relatively unstructured and therefore difficult to apply (Hauch et al., 2017; Ruby & Brigham, 1997; Vrij, 2005, 2016). Many studies have addressed the evidentiary power of CBCA, both in experiments and field studies, applied by trained and naïve experts, with and without VC. Overall, the accuracy is approximately 70% (Oberlader et al., 2016; Ruby & Brigham, 1997; Vrij, 2005). This is quite impressive, compared to other lie detection tools. However, it is arguably insufficient for practical application, given the 30% false conclusions. Here, it is important to distinguish scientific significance from diagnostic application in individual cases. Indeed, several authors advice against practical application of CBCA (see Hauch et al., 2017; Oberlader et al., 2016; Ruby & Brigham, 1997; Vrij, 2005).

Some limitations in the application of CBCA may suppress the accuracy of the instrument, and conversely, solving these limitations may increase accuracy. First, it is unclear when a testimony meets a particular criterion. For example, when is a testimony rich in detail (number 3)? One way to increase inter-rater reliability is to score each criterion on a scale from 0 through 2. However, there will always be a subjective component in the rating of criteria. Second, that subjectivity may be reduced if the expert were to compare the testimony subjected to his judgement with a "baseline" testimony given by the same witness. Third, it is unclear how many criteria need to be scored positively in order for a testimony to be considered valid. For example, if each criterion indeed were scored on a scale from 0 through 2, the total score would range between 0 and 38. But then still, it is unclear how high a testimony needs to score to be labelled valid. This cut-off score is particularly difficult to determine, because the CBCA criteria differ in nature. For example, many testimonies will not meet number 19 (specific details that can only be reported by a child witness if he actually witnessed the incident). Thus, this criterion is in practice rather seldom, and therefore not so useful. However, at the same time, if a testimony does include a unique detail, this same criterion instantly becomes extremely diagnostic. Hence, the presence of some criteria is not necessary but sufficient, whereas the presence of others (e.g., number 1, the logical structure) is necessary but not sufficient. So far, it seems that practicing legal psychologists as well as researchers make up their own decision rules, that mostly share the necessity of sufficing the first three criteria, combined with two or more (random) others (see Ruby & Brigham, 1997; Vrij, 2005). Given the difficulty of reaching consensus on a generally applicable cut-off score due to the different nature of the criteria, some authors (e.g., Hauch et al., 2017) argue against the use of total CBCA scores altogether. Fourth, whereas SVA, including CBCA, was originally meant to be applied to younger children's testimonies in sexual abuse cases, it is currently applied much broader, to older, even adult witnesses and other than abuse cases. Theoretically, this broad application will cause the technique to loose selectivity, that is, fabricated testimonies will be labelled as truthful. Finally, it is important to keep in mind that CBCA aims at distinguishing true from deceitful testimonies. CBCA is not sensitive to false testimonies based on false memories. Note that if the witness has a false memory, he is not lying, in that he lacks a deliberate motive to give a false testimony. Not all falsity is based on lies. In the words of Volbert and Steller: ‘CBCA characteristics … would seem to be less appropriate for distinguishing between truthful reports and accounts based on false memories’ (2014, p. 215), and: ‘If the fabrication hypothesis is falsified because of high content quality, this does not necessarily confirm the veracity of the testimony. As pointed out above, it is also necessary to test whether it could be based on a false memory’ (p. 214), and finally: ‘To examine the hypothesis that a statement is based on a false memory, it is necessary to focus on the way in which the statement has emerged and evolved’ (p. 207). Particularly, in the current case, the appropriate alternative hypothesis may be that the two women were not necessarily lying, but had developed false memories of the abuse.

In conclusion, while CBCA has a socially recommendable, and theoretically acceptable basis, its accuracy is impressive, with on average 70% (compared to 50% chance level), employing only a written testimony. Nonetheless, to actually uphold this accuracy rate (which is in fact low for application in individual cases), the legal psychologist should be considerate in using CBCA, and be aware of its limitations. A routine application of CBCA, without further academic thinking, can be quite problematic for the victim and suspect, but also for legal psychology as a mature discipline. Volbert and Steller (2014, p. 208) argue: ‘a non-critical application of CBCA may well lead to a false result in these cases’. They add that components of the VC are a crucial part of validity assessment: ‘the central diagnostic question when performing a credibility assessment in a single case is whether this particular witness could have or would have produced this testimony on this particular alleged event if it were not based on real experience’ (2014, p. 212).

Notably, in recent years, theory and findings regarding the detailedness (e.g., number 3 in CBCA) of truthful and false testimonies has evolved. The crucial idea in the verifiability approach is that counting the number of details may not always suffice to discriminate truthful and deceitful narratives. This is so because liars sometimes realise that increasing the number of details in their testimony will increase credibility. However, increasing details makes it more difficult to memorise the false narrative, and will thus decrease consistency which is bad for credibility. To escape this dilemma, liars may seek refuge in a ‘keep it simple’ strategy. Note that some details are easier to remember than others. For example, some details are actually simply common knowledge details. Likewise, self-handicapping details and irrelevant peripheral details are also fruitful to include in false narratives. By contrast, verifiable details (i.e., details that can theoretically be checked by third parties) and complications (unnecessary details that complicate reproduction of the narrative) will not be favoured by liars. These will appear, by contrast, in the narratives of truth-tellers, because truth-tellers are guided by a ‘tell it all’ strategy. In a handful of studies, truthful accounts have been documented to include more verifiable details than false accounts (Nahari & Vrij, 2014; Nahari et al., 2014). Some authors even argue that the absolute number of details should no longer be used as a sharp enough truth indicator. More fine graining indicators have been forwarded, such as the proportion of complications (complicating details/(complications + common knowledge details + self-handicapping details); see Nahari et al., 2019). Interestingly, a recent study by Verschuere et al. (2023) indicates that simply looking at detailedness yields accuracy rates similar to CBCA and the verifiability approach, after all.

5.2 Recovered Memories

If we are to take the allegation of the two women seriously, while abandoning the one-dimensional approach of CBCA and taking an analysis of competing hypotheses approach (cf. Heuer, 1999) instead, we first have to consider what is needed in the primary hypothesis. To start, the abuse was repressed by the two women. That is, they somehow completely forgot that it had happened, for years. Repression is strongly associated with the psychodynamic view forwarded by Sigmund Freud (1856–1939) who was actually a psychiatrist, but is considered a founding father of contemporary psychology. Freud has published a lot, in many different outlets such as (initially unpublished) letters to colleagues, books, and essays. There are at least three consistent themes in his work (e.g., Freud, 1910). First, Freud believed that all individuals have to go through five predetermined developmental stages in order to reach a sane mature mental state: The oral (age 0–1), anal (1–3), phallic (3–6), latent (7–11), and genital (11 <) phase. In all stages, the mental energy (*Lebenstrieb*) is remarkably consistently directed at the pertinent body parts. Going through all stages successfully is not always easy. For example, one can get stuck in a stage and the development arrests (fixation), or one can even fall back to a previously completed stage (regression). A second recurring theme is that in Freud's vision, the human mental system can actually be subdivided in two different ways. The first division is based on the guiding principles. The *Ich* is guided by the reality principle, the *Überich* is guided by morality, and the *Es* is guided by pleasure. These three systems are likely to get into conflict, because pleasure and morality do not always go hand in hand. The second division is between conscious and unconscious processing (and in some publications even a subconscious that functions in between). The two divisions are tied asymmetrically in that Überich and Es are almost completely unconscious, while Ich is partly conscious. In fact, Freud argued that most mental activity occurs outside our conscious awareness. The third recurring theme is that of the defence mechanisms. Ich, having a fulltime job reconciling conflicting input from Überich and Es, meanwhile trying to adapt to external reality, has numerous defence mechanisms at its disposal to keep up appearances. Notably, these defences are oftentimes unconscious. Best known are displacement, dictating that we can inhibit unwanted emotional reactions and transfer them onto another target later on (e.g., being furious at one's boss, but not telling him, while later being unkind to one's housemates), and projection (i.e., attributing some of one's own unwanted emotions to someone else). Given that all defences have in common that some part of reality is distorted or pushed outside of consciousness, repression (i.e., the motivated removal of unwanted impulses and memories from consciousness) is considered to be the mother of all defences.

It should be noted that Freud, being a psychiatrist, based his insights into the human psyche largely on his encounters with psychiatric patients. Given that individuals are, in the psychodynamic vision, expected to not have good self-insight, because most of the psychological processes occur outside conscious awareness, psychotherapists need to employ ingenious instruments to discover the underlying causes of current psychiatric symptoms. Hence, dream interpretation, free association, and hypnosis are some of the techniques used by psycho-analytic therapists. These techniques try to evade conscious reactions in order to reach the unconscious. Therefore, these techniques are referred to as indirect or projective techniques.

Looking back at Freud's work from a contemporary viewpoint, several critiques are in place. First, it is depressing that in the psychodynamic approach, all individuals are bound to get into psychological problems, if not because of flawed personality development, then because of conflicts between mature personality structures. Second, in the psychodynamic view, the majority of important mental activity occurs unconsciously. Thus, our conscious perception of ourselves and our environment is not much more than a superfluous side effect of the truly important processes occurring unconsciously. Third, Freud was a productive writer, but he sometimes contradicts his own prior work. For example in *The Aetiology of Hysteria* (1896/1959a), Freud explains his trauma and repression hypothesis which was based on his treatment of 18 patients. These patients subjected themselves to his treatment because of various hysterical complaints (i.e., anxieties). While they initially did not mention this, Freud discovered through projective techniques that they had had premature sexual encounters. The patients did not remember such abuse consciously, but Freud derived the occurrences from his diagnostic processes. Apparently, the abuse had been repressed into unconsciousness. Freud concluded that the 'hysterical symptoms are derivatives of memories operating unconsciously'. Strikingly, 9 years later in *My views on the part played by sexuality in the etiology of the neurosis* (1905/1959b), he withdraws his trauma and repression hypothesis and replaces it with a conflict theory. He now claims that the patients had not been abused, but their memories of the abuse were the result of internal conflict. Thus, the patients had developed false memories. In his words: 'I overestimated the frequency of these occurrences … I was not able to discriminate between the deceptive memories and actual happenings'. This turn is remarkable. While the patients had not mentioned the abuse but were informed about it by Freud himself, Freud later 'accused' them of having deceptive memories. Notably, many contemporary psychodynamic psychologists refuse to accept that Freud retracted his trauma and repression hypothesis. They believe that Freud published his 1905 paper merely for social-political reasons. It is believed that the (rich and influential) parents of the 18 patients confronted Freud with the curious outcome of his therapeutic experimentation (being that their children now falsely accused them of abuse), in reaction to which Freud retracted this theory just to remain at good terms with his cohabitants in Vienna (see Bowers & Farvolden, 1996). A fourth remark concerning Freud's work is actually not a critique. The original German texts by Freud are interesting, if not as a source of psychological theory, then as a souvenir of a past era. The work is also flooded with humour. Unfortunately, the English translations of Freud's work are at some points not completely adequate. For example, some of the typical German expressions (e.g., Ich, Überich, Es, Lebenstrieb, and Todestrieb) have been translated with Latin phrases (Ego, Superego, Id, Libido, and Thanatos) that sound much more serious. Much of the humour in Freud's original German writings is completely lacking from the English translations. A final remark is that Freud's way of developing theory is inadequate when judged by standards that have by now become virtually generally accepted in academic psychology.

So while there is little sound theoretical ground for the concept of repression, there may be other reasons for a recollection to become 'lost' for some time. One option would be that people may consciously try to suppress unwanted memories (whereas repression is supposed to occur without conscious efforts). However, in their classic study, Wegner et al. (1987) found that participants were not even able to avoid thoughts of a white bear for 5 min. Further, such suppression attempts turned out to have a rebound effect in that later on, more white bear intrusions occurred. In this line of reasoning, if people are generally not even able to suppress a discrete neutral thought, why would we be equipped with the capacity to suppress elaborate traumatic memories. However, Wegner et al. (1996) also found that the result of suppressing elaborate memories is that some parts that are suppressed will paradoxically be well remembered, but others less so, resulting in a decreased memory for the overall order of sequences. Similar findings (i.e., suppression attempts resulting in superior memory for some parts and inferior memory for others) have been observed with adapted research paradigms such as think-no-think, and retrieval-induced forgetting (Anderson & Green, 2001). In all, the research findings do not approach the washing away of complete memories as is needed in the original Freudian view on recovered memories.

A serious possibility for memories to become lost is simple forgetting (Schacter, 1999). That requires that we accept that even traumatic incidents can be forgotten (Kihlstrom, 2002). Whereas that might be difficult to appreciate, there is evidence to suggest that even traumatic incidents are not immune to forgetting. Wagenaar and Groeneweg (1990) reported a field study on traumatic memory. Background of this study was a Dutch prison camp (camp Erika) during World War II that shared characteristics with a concentration camp. Survivors of this camp were interviewed at the end of the war (1943–1948), and again after 40 years, between 1984 and 1987. Particularly, witnesses gave incriminating evidence against a fellow prisoner, Mar(t)inus de Rijke, who was made Kapo according to Nazi law. In all, 72 camp survivors were interviewed, some of them twice, with an interval of about 40 years. From these data, the authors concluded that the camp survivors had fairly consistent recollections of the maltreatments by de Rijke, but at the same time, they had forgotten quite some details. For example, some maltreated respondents (i.e., 8%) had forgotten de Rijke's name, or could not recognize him (i.e., 20%). Some of them even forgot having been maltreated or having been witness to murder. The authors conclude that 'intensity of experiences is not a sufficient safeguard against forgetting' (p. 77). More recently, Engelhard et al. (2008) tested the consistency of memories of 133 infantry troopers of their 4 months stay in Iraq in 2004. The soldiers were interviewed twice, after 5 and 15 months after returning from the mission. On both occasions, respondents were asked whether or not they had experienced any of 22 specific events during their military mission. Interestingly, while respondents were consistent in some respects, there were also remarkable inconsistencies. Table 5.1 presents examples of the 22 specific experiences, including the number of respondents who answered consistently and inconsistently at 5 and 15 months.

As can be seen, the percentages of participants who endorsed events inconsistently were sometimes quite remarkable. Indeed, on average over the 22 items, 17.5% of participants answered inconsistently. It can also be seen that while forgetting (yes to no changes) was prevalent, distortions/confabulations (no to yes changes) were virtually equally prevalent. Given that the ground truth is unknown to us, it can obviously not be concluded whether an inconsistency represents a flaw or an improvement. In total, the 133 soldiers made 259 negative changes (yes to no), and 249 positive changes (no to yes alteration). Again, these findings seem to illustrate that the intensity of experiences is no safeguard against forgetting or distortion.

Under the recovered memories hypothesis, the recollection must not only be lost for a prolonged period of time, it must remain unaltered during that period. Particularly, if it serves as evidence in a criminal trial, it must have high accuracy. While crucial and discrete information can be retained very long if not lifelong (Schmidt et al., 2000), there is reason to argue that complex memories do at least fade over time, even if they are remembered. Johnson et al. (1988) gave 72 undergraduates 4 differential memory assignments: They had to think of a recent social event, library visit or dentist visit, or of such an event in their childhood. Also, they had to think of a (recent or childhood) dream, fantasy, of unfulfilled intention. In all cases, participants rated their mental representation on 39 characteristics on a scale from 1 through 7. Johnson et al. used the scores on the so-called Memory

Table 5.1 Number of respondents ($N = 133$) who were consistent or inconsistent in their memory of a military mission, after 5 versus 15 months (Engelhard et al., 2008)

	Consistent		Inconsistent		Change %
	No-No	Yes-Yes	Yes-No	No-Yes	
Seeing dead or injured non-Dutch soldiers	79	16	22	16	29%
Seeing dead or injured Dutch soldiers	55	52	13	13	20%
Witnessing an explosion	20	90	14	9	17%
Witnessing violence	15	100	13	5	14%
Being shot at	33	75	6	19	19%
Being injured due to an assault	109	5	14	5	14%
Being sexually harassed	116	3	11	3	11%
Fearing to be taken hostage	16	88	18	18	27%

Characteristics Questionnaire (MCQ) to compare the different mental representations. The representations did not differ on all characteristic, but generally, memories for actually perceived events scored higher than those for imagined events. Likewise, recent memories scored higher than distant memories. Hence, it can be argued that old memories fade away into imagination-like representations. The MCQ items that turned out to differentiate memories for perceived and imagined events (and in some cases recent and childhood memories) are displayed in Table 5.2. Note that the (39) MCQ items are sometimes clustered into a handful of higher order criteria such as clarity, sensory information, context, thoughts and feelings, and intensity (e.g., Suengas & Johnson, 1988). It is believed that we (implicitly) use these characteristics when differentiating between actual events and imagined events (i.e., reality monitoring; RM). However, given that memories for actual distant events become similar to memories for imagined events, we will sometimes make mistakes, and confuse real events and imaginations. Hence, generally, our source monitoring (i.e., attributing our memories to the correct source, whether external or internal) capacity is limited.

Curiously, the MCQ is also advocated to be a useful verbal lie detection tool with accuracy equal to CBCA (Masip et al., 2005). The 39 items are then oftentimes

Table 5.2 MCQ scores (1–7) significantly differentiating real and imagined, and/or recent and distant mental representations (Johnson et al., 1988)

	Recent event	Recent imagination	Childhood event	Childhood imagination
Visual details	6.0	5.1	5.2	4.6
Sound	4.7	3.1	3.8	3.4
Smell	3.0	1.8	2.3	1.9
Taste	3.1	1.6	2.5	1.3
Complexity	2.4	3.4	2.8	3.3
Realism	6.4	5.0	5.8	3.9
Location	6.6	5.5	6.2	5.8
Setting	6.0	4.9	5.8	5.7
Spatial arrangement of objects	6.1	4.5	5.0	4.7
Time	5.9	4.0	4.0	4.0
Year	6.6	4.9	4.1	3.3
Season	6.1	4.8	3.8	3.7
Day	4.8	2.9	2.6	2.1
Hour	5.1	2.9	3.2	3.0
Emotional tone	5.5	4.5	4.8	4.5
Seeming implications	3.1	4.8	3.6	3.4
Intensity	4.4	5.4	4.8	5.0
Prior events	4.7	3.1	2.7	2.5
Posterior events	4.9	3.1	3.1	2.5
Covert rehearsal	3.3	4.5	3.0	3.5

clustered in to the following of which the first five characteristics are considered to indicate truthfulness, whereas the last indicates deceitfulness.

1. Contextual information (e.g., space and time references)
2. Sensory information (e.g., shapes, colours)
3. Semantic information (e.g., verbal interactions)
4. Emotional information
5. Clarity, vividness, realism, reconstructability
6. Cognitive operations (e.g., guessing and out loud reconstructing, rather than reporting straight forwardly from memory)

Compared to CBCA, RM has some advantages. It does not require extensive and expensive training, it is not limited in age (although increases in age go hand-in-hand with higher scores, regardless of truth status; Masip et al., 2005), nor in applicable crimes: It can be employed regardless of crime type. Given the theoretical background of the RM approach, it can be expected that RM is not only applicable in situations in which the question is whether the witness or suspect is lying, but also if the alternative scenario implies that he might be mistaken.

The final assumption we must be willing to make in the recovered memories hypothesis is that the long-lost memory can be recovered during therapy without it being altered. It is difficult to imagine how a therapist can make a patient realise that there was a traumatic incident in the past, when that patient has absolutely no recollection thereof. Once the therapist finds out that this is so, he must at the very least make a remark such as 'I have seen many patients with complaints similar to yours, and they turned out to have experienced and completely forgotten a traumatic event in their younger years'. However, from a legal psychology viewpoint, such a remark is suggestive and would make it impossible to claim that the patient recovered the memory completely independently, and thus, it would suppress authenticity and validity.

In sum, the recovered memory hypothesis requires a few bold assumptions, that legal psychologists are not always willing to make, unlike psychotherapists. Hence, there is a strong difference of opinion between science-oriented and therapy-oriented psychologists. The latter regularly see patients who recover lost memories of trauma, whereas the former make critical remarks about such recovery. The debate about recovered memories has at times been so intense that it was referred to as a memory war, that raged in the late twentieth century, but may still not be over yet (Dodier, 2019; Karon & Widener, 1997; Loftus & Davis, 2006; Loftus & Ketcham, 1994; Otgaar et al., 2019; Patihis et al., 2014).

5.3 Clinical Versus Legal Psychology

It must be acknowledged that clinical and legal psychology differ in a few fundamental respects, which may account for the vastly different views on recovered memories. For example, clinical and counselling psychologists adhere to several professional attitudes that serve well in a therapeutic setting but are detrimental in a legal context. Greenberg and Shuman (1997) discussed 10 differences between clinical and forensic roles. These differences are so fundamental that Richards et al. (2015) refer to the intertwinement of the different roles as a role bias. One difference is that for clinical psychologists, the client himself is the commissioning party (albeit oftentimes indirectly via the company that the psychologist works for), whereas in a forensic context, the judge or lawyer is the commissioning party. Consequently, whereas in a clinical context, there is a therapist-client confidentiality, the allegiance of the forensic psychologist lies with the judge. Next, whereas a clinical psychologist is expected to display an empathic attitude, the forensic psychologist needs to be more distant, neutral, and detached. Obviously, clinical roles require different capabilities (treatment techniques) than do forensic roles (e.g., evaluation, diagnostics). The goal of a therapeutic cooperation between the clinical psychologist and the client is to improve the client's wellbeing, whereas the goal of the forensic psychologist is factual diagnostics. In other words, the therapeutic role is client-centred, whereas the forensic role is truth-centred. In the light of this, factual scrutinization is less in clinical roles than in forensic roles. For example, if a client is referred to a psychotherapist by his physician for the treatment of Post-Traumatic Stress Disorder (PTSD), the psychologist will take the PTSD and the client's narratives about it as a starting point. The psychologist will not ask for proof of the traumatisation that caused the PTSD. Neither will he start a police investigation. That would be at odds with therapist-client confidentiality. In essence, clinical psychologists have a professionally dictated truth bias. This is deeply at odds with a forensic context in which the client (or rather, the object of investigation) cannot always be expected to be sincere, or even to be willing to cooperate. Whereas the regular client in clinical psychological contexts approaches the therapist because he needs help with his problem, the suspect or witness do not necessarily come voluntarily, do not (believe that they) have a problem, and have nothing to gain from their encounter with the psychologist. Rassin and Merckelbach (1999) described another difference, namely that between the primary error detection and minimisation in clinical and forensic contexts. For the clinician, the worst possible mistake is to miss an illness (i.e., a false negative), especially if the illness is severe, and the treatment relatively free of side effects and thus harmless (but see Lilienfeld, 2007, for not so harmless psychological interventions). So, if a client claims to have complaints caused by a traumatic experience, it is worse if the psychologist does not diagnose PTSD, while the client's complaints are genuine, than to diagnose PTSD even though the client's complaints are false or exaggerated. However, in a forensic context, the priorities are reversed. Here, a false positive is the primary error, because, if the witness (victim) is diagnosed with PTSD although he was not actually the victim of trauma, this false positive diagnosis may reflect on the perceived likelihood that the suspect is guilty of doing something traumatising to the victim. Thus, a false positive diagnosis in the clinical context is not all to detrimental, but if it will transpose to a false positive in the legal context, it will become detrimental, because it harms the presumption of innocence. Boeschen et al. (1998) distinguish five levels of expert testimony regarding PTSD. The first level occurs when the defence seeks to discredit a witness (a traumatised victim) by stressing the unusual behaviour of the witness (e.g., emotionality, irrationality). At this level, the psychologist may explain the witness' unusual behaviour in terms of consequences of traumatisation. At the second level, a clinical psychologist may testify about diagnostic criteria of PTSD in general. At level three, the expert testifies about the consistency of the witness' behaviour with PTSD symptoms. The fourth level is that the expert testifies in court that the witness suffers from PTSD. This level is, according to the authors, not recommendable, even if the witness gives permission to disclose this diagnosis. This is so because, while the diagnostic specificity of PTSD measures is considerable with a false positive rate of approximately 10–20%, and thus sufficient for clinical purposes, it falls short for application in a legal, fact-finding context. At the fifth level, the clinician would not only disclose that the witness suffers from PTSD, but also claim that what the witness testifies about the alleged trauma, must therefore be considered valid. Shuman et al. (1998) discuss a final reason for clinical psychologists not to let themselves be lured into the role of expert witness. That is, if the psychologist indeed discloses everything he has documented concerning his client, during court sessions, the client may be exposed to the psychologist's observations of him with which he disagrees. If so, this will harm the fruitful cooperation from then on. Alternatively, if the psychologist chooses to withhold certain details, the judge may get a dishonest impression of the psychologist, and that may harm the witness' case. Shuman et al. (1998) conclude: 'Either way, therapy loses' (p. 521). They wonder whether treating mental health professionals should be barred from testifying in court all together. Against this background, Zajac et al. (2013) propose quite strict thresholds for psychologists to serve as expert witness in sexual abuse court cases: 'At the minimum these experts will have earned a PhD in psychology or a related discipline, hold a position at a research institution, and have published a significant number of empirical papers in internationally recognised peer-reviewed journals (for the most part, conference presentations or posters are no substitute for peer-reviewed journal publications). It is also our view that people whose primary occupation is clinical practice are not automatically qualified to give evidence on human memory, even if they have published the occasional paper' (p. 615).

5.4 The Alternative Hypothesis

Under the alternative hypothesis, the two women in this case must somehow have developed intense false memories that made them become convinced to have been abused in the past even though they were not. As counterintuitive as that may seem, there is indeed some evidence that people can fall prey to intense false memories, and that the risk of that may run in the dozens of percentages. Below, a handful of relevant scientific studies will be discussed.

A first mechanism through which false memories can develop is the mixture of separate recollections into one intertwined version. In the previously mentioned classic study by Carmichael et al. (1932), participants were shown ambiguous pictures that were accompanied by verbal descriptions. Notably, each ambiguous picture was accompanied by one of two competing descriptions. Next, participants were instructed to reproduce the pictures regardless of the verbal descriptions. Remarkably, the reproductions were typically influenced by the verbal descriptions. Examples of this phenomenon are presented in Fig. 5.1. Apparently, the visual memory of the pictures was affected by the verbal memory. This effect is referred to as the verbal labelling or verbal overshadowing effect.

Another pathway to false memories that runs spontaneously and unconsciously is by association. Take the following word list: Note, sound, piano, sing, radio, band, melody, horn, concert, instrument, symphony, jazz, orchestra, art, rhythm. When recalling this list, one might through association easily remember the word music, even though it was not in the original list. Roediger and McDermott (1995) had participants study several word lists in which associated words (critical lures) were omitted. While on average 65% of the presented words were recalled immediately after exposure, so was 40% of the critical lures. In a subsequent recognition test, in which the critical lures were included, 81% of the lures was recognised, on average. This Deese Roediger McDermott (DRM) effect illustrates a source monitoring flaw, or misattribution (Schacter, 1999): We are unable to differentiate between a witnessed stimulus, and an internally generated associate. Another illustration of misattribution is the false fame effect. In a typical study, participants are presented with a list of names of unknown people. Twenty-four hours later, they are

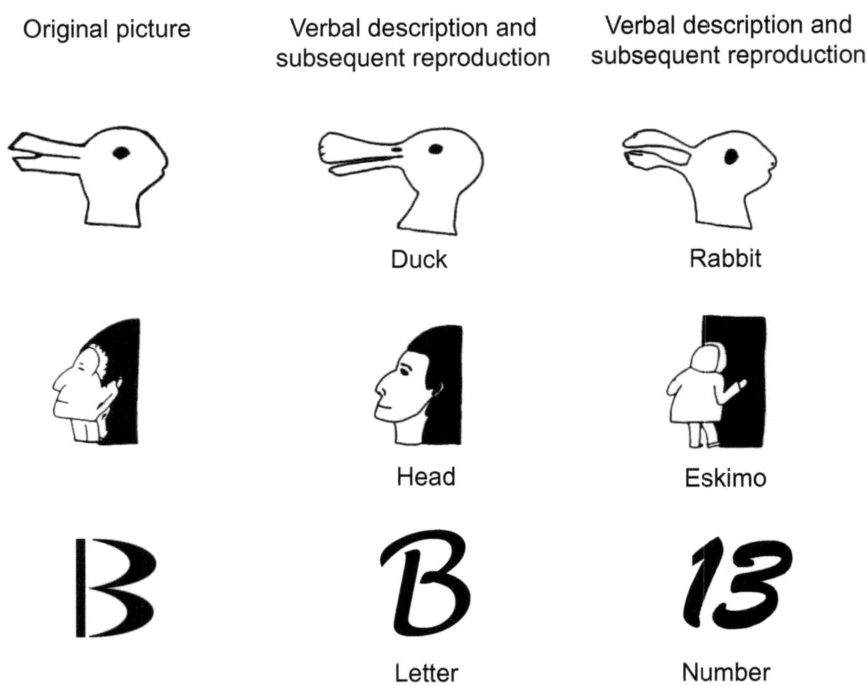

Fig. 5.1 Examples after the Carmichael et al. (1932) verbal labelling study

asked to indicate whether or not these (and other) names are famous. Strikingly, a significant part of the unknown names is then identified as a famous name. Apparently, people misinterpret the familiarity of the names (they saw them yesterday) for fame. Given that this effect occurs overnight, it has been argued to be a sleeper effect (cf. an unconscious increase of strength due to merely passing of time; see Jacoby et al., 1989).

Yet another paradigm used in experiments to illustrate flaws in source attribution, ultimately resulting in false memories, is imagination inflation. Thomas and Loftus (2002) conjured up 54 small behavioural actions, some of which are regular (e.g., flipping a coin), while others are bizarre (e.g., kissing a magnifying glass). Two hundred and ten undergraduates were invited to carry out 18 of these actions, to imagine doing them (18), or were given no instruction, even though the materials for these remaining 18 actions were laid out on the table. The next day, the participants underwent an imagination session during which actions were imagined zero, one, or five times (for 7 s each). Two weeks later, participants were asked to indicate for all 54 actions whether they had performed them during the first session, or merely imagined them, or neither. For actions that had actually been carried out, source monitoring was fairly accurate with on average 78% of the actions never imagined during session 2 recognised, 84% of the carried-out during session 1 and imagined once during session 2 actions recognised, and 85% of the actions imagined five times. However, the findings for actions merely imagined in session 1, or not presented at all during session 1, recognition patterns were similar and largely dependent on instructions during session 2. In absence of imagination during session 2, approximately 3.5% of these (not carried out) actions were mistakenly recognised as actions actually carried out. When imagined once during session 2, 19.5% was mistaken for actual actions, and when imagined five times during session 2, 23.5% of the actions were mistakenly recognised during session 3 as actions actually carried out. These findings again illustrate that source monitoring is fragile and susceptible to mistakes (see also Loftus, 2003).

The examples discussed so far refer to spontaneous false memory development. In the current case, such processes may occur (under the alternative hypothesis, that is) when the women merely thought about the abuse, possibly advised to do so by therapists. But there is also a possibility that they were exposed to some, even minor, suggestive questions from each other or third parties like therapists. That would introduce an additional possibility for false memory elicitation. The detrimental effect of suggestion on memory and subsequent narrative production has been documented in manifold. A hallmark study is the one by Loftus and Palmer (1974). These authors showed 45 undergraduates one of seven short (5–30 s) film fragments depicting a car crash. Next, they asked participants to estimate the speed of the cars ('About how fast were the cars going when they *contacted* each other?'). Crucially, in parallel versions of the questionnaire, the verb contact was replaced by hit, bumped, collided, or smashed. Strikingly, the mean estimated speed was strongly affected by this one verb. That is, while the estimated speed was 31.8 mph in the contact condition, in the hit, bumped, collided and smashed conditions, the means were 34, 38.1, 39.3, and 40.8 mph. Given that the authors used different film fragments in which the cars drove at different speeds, it is impossible to determine the accuracy of these estimates. Nevertheless, it is obvious that the estimates were affected by the precise wording of the pertinent question. In their second study, 150 students watched a short film of a car crash and were again asked to estimate the speed of the cars. For some respondents, the question included the word hit, for others the word smashed. Respective estimates were 8 and 10.46 mph. Next, they were asked whether they had seen any broken wind shields in the film (whereas in reality, there were no broken windows). Fourteen percent of the participants who had previously estimated the cars' speed when they hit, now mistakenly believed to have seen shattered glass, compared to 32% in the smashed condition. Hence, the findings clearly illustrate the effect of leading/suggestive questions.

In a comparable study, Crombag et al. (1996) asked 193 respondents whether they had seen live film footage of a plane crash on October 4, 1992. In this crash, a cargo plane crashed into a building. In reality, film footage of the crash does not exist. No less than 107 (i.e., 55%) respondents answered this suggestive question affirmatively. These respondents were subsequently asked whether they remembered seeing fire break out at impact, or after a delay. Sixty three of them (59%) remembered seeing the fire occur at impact, 24 (23%) thought they had seen a short delay, and 20 (18%) testified they did not remember. In a replication in a sample of 93 law undergraduates, 66% misremembered seeing the film, and again, a significant proportion of them answered detailed questions about the occurrence of fire (67%), the position of the plane (horizontally versus vertically; 77%), and about what happened to the plane after impact (e.g., disintegration, falling on the ground, or remaining stuck in the building; 49%). In an overview of studies employing this crashing memories paradigm, it was found that on average 45% of participants will accept the suggestion of the non-existent film, and 24% will falsely remember details from that film (Rassin, 2022).

Meanwhile, it seems that false memories can be tenacious, intense and lively, and resistant to falsification (Scoboria et al., 2017). For example, McNally et al. (2004) confronted 10 individuals who had (false) memories of being abducted by aliens with transcripts of their abduction and with transcripts of actually experienced stressful events unrelated to alien abduction. The authors found that the individuals responded equally emotionally to the abduction transcripts as to the stressful transcripts, not only by self-report, but also as measured with physiological measures. Likewise, Lipinski and Pope (1994) described cases of patients who were treated for PTSD, while their traumatic flashbacks later turned out to be obsessive imageries. These findings illustrate that false memories can be quite vivid, intense, tenacious, and even physically arousing. Further, research has also shown that false memories of repeated events can be implanted in laboratory settings (Calado et al., 2021).

In short, it seems to be possible to develop false memories even of traumatic experiences. Not only Freud encountered 18 patients with such false memories, but in controlled laboratory settings, false memories seem to be elicitable relatively easily. The strength, intensity, and content of the memories does not seem to be a reliable cue to distinguish factual from false memories.

5.5 How the Case Ended

In my report, I warned the judge for the possibility that the allegations may fit well in an alternative hypothesis that revolves around false memory development caused by actively searching for traumatic experiences in the distant past to explain the current unhappiness (but see Gewehr et al., 2021, for the argument that old allegations are not necessarily false), suggestive interventions and imagery (as is to be expected in psychotherapies such as hypnotherapy and EMDR; Otgaar et al., 2021), and joint efforts at memory work such as visiting the suspect's house. That is not the same as saying that the memories were false.

Eventually the court acquitted the suspect. The judge found the allegations unreliable, particularly because of the long retention interval, the fact that the memories had been repressed and recovered in therapy, the fact that the women spoke of their memories in terms of flashbacks and dream-like recollections, and the fact that there was an increment in the content of the allegations (i.e., they got worse in the course of various interviews), and they were thus inconsistent.

References

Anderson, M. C., & Green, C. (2001). Suppressing unwanted memories by executive control. *Nature, 410*, 366–369.

Boeschen, L. E., Sales, B. D., & Koss, M. P. (1998). Rape trauma experts in the courtroom. *Psychology, Public Policy, and Law, 4*, 414–432.

Bowers, K. S., & Farvolden, P. (1996). Revisiting a century-old Freudian slip: From suggestion disavowed to the truth repressed. *Psychological Bulletin, 119*, 355–380.

Calado, B., Luke, T. J., Connolly, D. A., Landstrom, S., & Otgaar, H. (2021). Implanting false autobiographical memories for repeated events. *Memory, 29*(10), 1320–1341.

Carmichael, L. C., Hogan, H. P., & Walter, A. A. (1932). An experimental study of the effect of language on the reproduction of visually perceived forms. *Journal of Experimental Psychology, 15*, 73–86.

Crombag, H. F. M., Wagenaar, W. A., & Van Koppen, P. J. (1996). Crashing memories and the problem of 'source monitoring'. *Applied Cognitive Psychology, 10*, 95–104.

Dodier, O. (2019). A bibliometric analysis of the recovered memory controversy in the 21st century. *Applied Cognitive Psychology, 33*(4), 571–584.

Engelhard, I. M., van den Hout, M. A., & McNally, R. J. (2008). Memory consistency for traumatic events in Dutch soldiers deployed to Iraq. *Memory, 16*, 3–9.

Freud. (1910). *Eine Kintheitserinnerung des Leonardo da Vinci.* W.W. Norton & Company.

Freud, S. (1959a). The aetiology of hysteria. In J. Riviere (red). *Sigmund Freud: Collected papers, Volume 1* (pp. 183–219). New York: Basic books.

Freud, S. (1959b). My views on the part of sexuality in the aetiology of the neurosis. In J. Riviere (red.). *Sigmund Freud: Collected papers, Volume 1* (pp. 272–283). New York: Basic Books.

Gewehr, E., Hensel, B., & Volbert, R. (2021). Predicting disclosure latency in substantiated cases of child sexual abuse. *Child Abuse & Neglect, 122*, 105346.

Greenberg, S. A., & Shuman, D. W. (1997). Irreconcilable conflict between therapeutic and forensic roles. *Professional Psychology: Research and Practice, 28*, 50–57.

Hauch, V., Sporer, S. L., Masip, J., & Blandón-Gitlin, I. (2017). Can credibility criteria be assessed reliably? A meta-analysis of criteria-based content analysis. *Psychological Assessment, 29*, 819–834.

Heuer, R. J. (1999). *Psychology of intelligence analyses*. CIA.

Jacoby, L. L., Kelley, C. M., Brown, J., & Jasechko, J. (1989). Becoming famous overnight: Limits on the ability to avoid unconscious influences of the past. *Journal of Personality and Social Psychology, 56*, 326–338.

Johnson, M. K., Foley, M. A., Suengas, A. G., & Raye, C. L. (1988). Phenomenal characteristics of memories for perceived and imagined autobiographical events. *Journal of Experimental Psychology: General, 117*, 371–376.

Karon, B. P., & Widener, A. J. (1997). Repressed memories and world war II: Lest we forget! *Professional Psychology: Research and Practice, 28*, 338–340.

Kihlstrom, J. F. (2002). No need for repression. *Trends in Cognitive Sciences, 6*, 502.

Lilienfeld, S. O. (2007). Psychological treatments that cause harm. *Perspectives on Psychological Science, 2*, 53–70.

Lipinski, J. F., & Pope, H. G. (1994). Do "flashbacks" represent obsessional imagery? *Comprehensive Psychiatry, 35*, 245–247.

Loftus, E. F. (2003). Make-believe memories. *American Psychologist, 58*, 867–873.

Loftus, E. F., & Davis, D. (2006). Recovered memories. *Annual Review of Clinical Psychology, 2*, 469–498.

Loftus, E. F., & Ketcham, K. (1994). *The myth of repressed memory: False memories and allegations of sexual abuse*. St. Martin's Press.

Loftus, E. F., & Palmer, J. C. (1974). Reconstruction of automobile destruction: An example of the interaction between language and memory. *Journal of Verbal Learning and Verbal Behavior, 13*, 585–589.

Masip, J. M., Sporer, S. L., Garrido, E., & Herrero, C. (2005). The detection of deception with the reality monitoring approach: A review of the empirical evidence. *Psychology, Crime & Law, 11*, 99–122.

McNally, R. J., Lasko, N. B., Clancy, S. A., Macklin, M. L., Pitman, R. K., & Orr, S. P. (2004). Psychophysiological responding during script-driven imagery in people reporting abduction by space aliens. *Psychological Science, 15*, 493–497.

Nahari, G., & Vrij, A. (2014). Can I borrow your alibi? The applicability of the verifiability approach to the case on an alibi witness. *Journal of Applied Research in Memory and Cognition, 3*, 89–94.

Nahari, G., Vrij, A., & Fisher, R. P. (2014). The verifiability approach: Countermeasures facilitate its ability to discriminate between truths and lies. *Applied Cognitive Psychology, 28*, 122–128.

Nahari, G., Ashkenazi, T., Fisher, R. P., Granhag, P. A., Hershkowitz, I., Masip, J., Meijer, E. H., Nisin, Z., Sarid, N., Taylor, P. J., Verschuere, B., & Vrij, A. (2019). 'Language of lies': Urgent issues and prospects in verbal lie detection research. *Legal and Criminological Psychology, 24*, 1–23.

Oberlader, V. A., Naefgen, C., Koppehele-Gossel, J., Quinten, L., Banse, R., & Schmidt, A. F. (2016). Validity of content-based techniques to distinguish true and fabricated statements: A meta-analysis. *Law and Human Behavior, 40*, 440–457.

Otgaar, H., Howe, M. L., Patihis, L., Merckelbach, H., Lynn, S. J., Lilienfeld, S. O., & Loftus, E. F. (2019). The return of the repressed: The persistent and problematic claims of long-forgotten trauma. *Perspectives on Psychological Science, 14*(6), 1072–1095.

Otgaar, H., Houben, S., Rassin, E., & Merckelbach, H. (2021). Memory and eye movement desensitization and reprocessing therapy: A potentially risky combination in the courtroom. *Memory, 29*, 1254–1262.

Patihis, L., Ho, L. Y., Tingen, I. W., Lilienfeld, S. O., & Loftus, E. F. (2014). Are the "memory wars" over? A scientist-practitioner gap in beliefs about memory. *Psychological Science, 25*, 519–530.

Rassin, E. (2022). Suggested false memories of a non-existent film: Forensically relevant individual differences in the *crashing memories* paradigm. *Memory, 30*(9), 1205–1211.

Rassin, E., & Merckelbach, H. (1999). The potential conflict between clinical and judicial decision making heuristics. *Behavioral Sciences & the Law, 17*, 237–248.

Richards, P. M., Geiger, J. A., & Tussey, C. M. (2015). The dirty dozen: 12 sources of bias in forensic neuropsychology with ways to mitigate. *Psychological Injury and Law, 8*, 265–280.

Roediger, H. L., & McDermott, K. B. (1995). Creating false memories: Remembering words not presented in lists. *Journal of Experimental Psychology: Learning, Memory and Cognition, 24*, 803–814.

Ruby, C. L., & Brigham, J. C. (1997). The usefulness of the criteria-based content analysis technique in distinguishing between truthful and fabricated allegations: A critical review. *Psychology, Public Policy, and Law, 3*, 705–737.

Schacter, D. L. (1999). The seven sins of memory. *American Psychologist, 54*, 182–203.

Schmidt, H. G., Peeck, V. H., Paas, F., & Van Breukelen, G. J. P. (2000). Remembering the street names of one's childhood neighbourhood: A study of very long-term retention. *Memory, 8*, 37–49.

Scoboria, A., Wade, K. A., Lindsay, D. S., Azad, T., Strange, D., Ost, J., & Hyman, I. E. (2017). A mega-analysis of memory reports from eight peer-reviewed false memory implantation studies. *Memory, 25*(2), 146–163.

Shuman, D. W., Greenberg, S., Heilbrun, K., & Foote, W. E. (1998). An immodest proposal: Should treating mental health professionals be barred from testifying about their patients? *Behavioral Sciences & the Law, 16*, 509–523.

Steller, M. & Köhnken, G. (1989). Criteria-based statement analysis: Credibility assessment of children's statements in sexual abuse cases. In D.C. Raskin (red.). *Psychological Methods for Investigating Evidence* (pp. 217–245). New York: Springer.

Suengas, A. G., & Johnson, M. K. (1988). Qualitative effects of rehearsal on memories for perceived and imagined complex events. *Journal of Experimental Psychology: General, 117*, 377–389.

Thomas, A. K., & Loftus, E. F. (2002). Creating bizarre false memories through imagination. *Memory & Cognition, 30*, 423–431.

Undeutsch, U. (1967). Beurteilung der Glaubhaftigkeit von Aussagen. In: U. Undeutsch (red.). *Handbuch der Psychologie, 11: Forensische Psychologie* (pp. 26–181). Göttingen: Hogrefe.

Verschuere, B., Lin, C. C., Huismann, S., Kleinberg, B., Willemse, M., Mei, C. J., & E., Van Goor, T., Löwy, L. H. S., Appiah, O. K. & Meijer, E. (2023). The use-the-best heuristic facilitates deception detection. *Nature Human Behaviour*. https://doi.org/10.1038/s41562-023-01556-2

Volbert, R., & Steller, M. (2014). Is this testimony truthful, fabricated, or based in false memory? Credibility assessment 25 years after Steller and Köhnken (1989). *European Psychologist, 19*, 207–220.

Vrij, A. (2005). Criteria-based content analysis: A qualitative review of the first 37 studies. *Psychology, Public Policy, and Law, 11*, 3–41.

Vrij, A. (2016). Baselining as a lie detection method. *Applied Cognitive Psychology, 30*, 1112–1119.

Wagenaar, W. A., & Groeneweg, J. (1990). The memory of concentration camp survivors. *Applied Cognitive Psychology, 4*(2), 77–87.

Wegner, D. M., Schneider, D. J., Carter, S. R., & White, T. L. (1987). Paradoxical effects of thought suppression. *Journal of Personality and Social Psychology, 53*, 5–13.

Wegner, D. M., Quillian, F., & Houston, C. (1996). Memories out of order: Thought suppression and the disassembly of remembered experience. *Journal of Personality and Social Psychology, 71*, 680–691.

Zajac, R., Garry, M., London, K., Goodyear-Smith, F., & Hayne, H. (2013). Misconceptions about childhood sexual abuse and child witnesses: Implications for psychological experts in the courtroom. *Memory, 21*, 608–617.

Chapter 6
Dissociation as a State of Reduced Consciousness

A middle-aged woman filed a complaint against a social worker in 2013. He was appointed as her guide in her reintegration trajectory somewhere around 2009. She was in this trajectory because she had been absent from work for a prolonged period. Her absence was caused by mental problems allegedly rooted in abuse in her childhood. In 2011, the social worker stopped working on the woman's case. However, she asked him for further contact outside their now ended formal working relationship. They kept in contact. This contact turned physical, and they had sexual intercourse multiple times, at the woman's home. The purpose of this sex was to suppress the intrusive reliving of her past traumatic abuse. At some point, the social worker ended the contact. Sometime later, she filed allegation for sexual abuse. She testified that during the sexual contacts, she was reliving past trauma, and in this dissociative state she was subconscious and thus not able to resist the suspect who then took advantage of her. The suspect testified that he enjoyed the sex, but its main purpose was always to help the woman, and he ended it after some time when he got bored and saw no progress in her recovery. The court asked two experts, me and Dr. Han Israels, for an opinion on the validity of the woman's allegation.

6.1 Laypeople's Strange Beliefs About Psychological Treatment

Under the primary hypothesis, the suspect took advantage of the victim who was unable to resist because of the dissociative state she was in. Under the alternative hypothesis, the sex happened with mutual consent. At closer inspection, the primary hypothesis illustrates a handful of weird assumptions that both the victim and the

ECLI:NL:GHARL:2018:8800

E. Rassin, *Case Studies in Legal Psychology*,
https://doi.org/10.1007/978-3-031-44931-4_6

suspect may have had concerning psychotherapy. Particularly, it seems as if they mixed up various concepts into a strange and non-existent compilation.

First, the woman referred to her dissociative state. Dissociation is complex because it refers to different phenomena. It can refer to a psychodynamic defensive reaction. In this definition, the psyche somehow manages to distract itself from an ongoing traumatic experience, in order to avoid painful emotions. In the words of Gershuny and Thayer: '… some kind of divided or parallel access to awareness in which two or more mental processes or contents are not associated or integrated, and awareness of one's emotions or thoughts are diminished and avoided' (1999, p. 637). Because this defensive reaction occurs during the traumatic experience, it is also known as peritraumatic dissociation. Subclinical manifestations of this type of dissociation are quite common. For example, when waking up in a strange bed (e.g., while on vacation or in a hospital), many people experience some kind of alienation, derealization, or depersonalization (American Psychiatric Association [APA], 2013). Moreover, this state can even be induced, for example by looking into a mirror for minutes (e.g., Brewin & Mersaditabari, 2013). Obviously, this state can be quite benign. It only becomes clinically relevant if it occurs often and causes stress. Dissociation can also refer to a clinical syndrome characterized by memory problems. In this definition, it is not only a psychodynamic reaction, but also the end result thereof, namely the loss of memory for the traumatic event that caused it. It is then referred to as dissociative amnesia. Some researchers have problems with this latter dynamic, even though it is currently an official diagnose in the Diagnostic and Statistical Manual of Mental Disorders (DSM; APA, 2013). The problem is that this concept requires that we are capable of shoving off complete experiences into unconsciousness. Hence, dissociation suffers the same critique as does repression (resulting in psychogenic amnesia), discussed in Chap. 5. In fact, Otgaar et al. (2019) argue that if we replace repression with dissociation in many papers in the memory wars, the same discussion is currently done all over. The only difference is that repression allegedly occurs after the trauma whereas dissociation does during. As with psychogenic amnesia due to repression, the evidence for dissociative amnesia largely rests on case studies (Mangiulli et al., 2022). Also similar to repression, there are some alternative accounts of dissociative amnesia. Kindt and van den Hout (2003) exposed 330 participants to an aversive film fragment, and asked them to concurrently complete a Peritraumatic Dissociative Experiences Questionnaire (PDEQ). Four hours later, participants completed metamemory items about their recollection of the film, as well as questions about the content of the film. Scores on the PDEQ did not correlate with performance on the content items, but did with the metamemory scale. That is, higher scores on dissociation were associated with a perceived fragmentation and deterioration of memory. Kindt and van den Hout conclude that '... dissociation induced memory fragmentation is confined to the realm of subjective experience and that dissociation may leave actual memory performance unaffected' (2003, p. 176).

Possibly the most rare and spectacular manifestation of dissociation is the Dissociative Identity Disorder (DID, APA, 2013). In this syndrome, dissociation will not only result in amnesia for the traumatic periods in which dissociation occurred, but also in the development of alternative personalities, alter egos. It is assumed that during traumatic experiences, the psyche creates an alternative consciousness that has to live through the trauma. Once the trauma is over, the original person returns but will suffer amnesia for the whole period during which the alter ego was active. In the words of the APA: 'Dissociative identity disorder is associated with overwhelming experiences, traumatic events, and/or abuse occurring in childhood' (2013, p. 294). Obviously, this can easily turn into a psychiatric disorder (if it is not already by definition), but it is also spectacular and it served as the starting point of literature (e.g., Jekyll and Hyde, the Hulk, Fight Club, Batman's Joker, to name a few). Strikingly, alter egos can be completely oblivious of each other's existence. To test this inter-identity amnesia, Huntjens et al. (2007) presented amnestic alter egos with separate word lists. They showed eight words (List A) to alter ego 1 of 19 DID patients with diagnosed inter-identity amnesia. Next, the patients switched identity to alter ego 2 (this switching is apparently under conscious control to some extent), and this alter ego was shown another list of eight words (List B). Two hours later, alter ego 2 underwent a recognition test in which they were shown 24 words. Of these, eight were from List B (these words should be recognized well), eight were from List A (these words should not be recognized because alter ego 2 was amnestic for alter ego 1's experiences), and eight were new, not previously shown words, to establish a base rate of false positives. For comparison purposes, the authors also included 25 healthy control participants who were instructed to recognize both word lists, and 25 healthy controls who were instructed to recognize words from List B and to simulate amnesia for the words from List A. The percentages of recognized words as function of sample and List are presented in Fig. 6.1. As can be seen, while simulators failed to successfully feign amnesia for List A, DID patients recognized too many words from List A to argue that alter ego 2 was indeed amnestic for the words shown to alter ego 1.

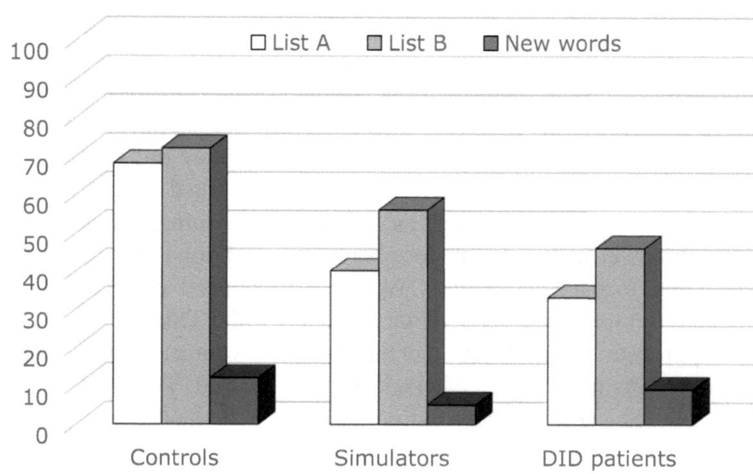

Fig. 6.1 Percentages of recognized words (Huntjens et al., 2007)

The findings by Huntjens et al. (2007) confirm that dissociative amnesia may not be at an objective level, but merely on a subjective, perceived level. Hence, the authors argue that the trauma model for dissociative amnesia should be replaced by a sociocognitive model. To date, there is still intense discussion as to which of these models deserve priority (e.g., Merckelbach & Patihis, 2018).

Regardless of the scientific discussion, the DSM (APA, 2013) does include dissociative symptoms that match those described by the woman in the current case. The symptoms of PTSD include 'recurrent, involuntary, and intrusive distressing memories of the traumatic event(s)', and 'dissociative reactions (e.g., flashbacks) in which the individual feels or acts as if the traumatic event(s) were recurring' (p. 271). The DSM also describes the dissociative trance 'characterized by an acute narrowing or complete loss of awareness of immediate surroundings that manifests as profound unresponsiveness of insensitivity to environmental stimuli' (p. 307).

A second assumption underlying the sexual relation between the woman in this case and her social worker is that she had to have sex as a therapeutic intervention. I understand that sex can be beneficial, if for no other reason because it can be a pleasant experience. There is an alternative therapeutic operationalization, namely that the woman wanted to expose herself to her traumatic memories so as to desensitize herself and make the negative emotions associated with the memories go extinct. Such exposure stems from behaviourism and is a strong therapeutic intervention (Eysenck, 1994). It is also a main component of the previously discussed EMDR.

Whereas so far, it might seem logical that the woman thought that having sex with her social worker and reliving past traumatic sexual experiences was a feasible therapeutic approach, below I will discuss the problems with this notion. First, pleasant and beneficial to mental health as it may be, therapists do not have sex with clients. At least not if they are serious psychotherapists. Moreso, in many legal systems sex between caregivers and caretakers is prohibited. If the sex was meant to somehow undo past abusive experiences by having pleasant sexual experiences, it is difficult to see why the woman would experience dissociative complaints during these new therapeutic sexual activities with the social worker. Dissociation occurs during traumatic events. By contrast, if the woman sought extinction of her aversion by repeated exposure to her traumatic memories, they should have concentrated on her aversive memories, flashbacks, and relivings, but they did not need to have actual sex simultaneously. Obviously, it would be a crooked idea to undergo new repeated traumatic sexual experiences as a means of exposure. As mentioned, exposure therapy is powerful, but one obvious boundary condition is that the stimulus we expose ourselves to is in fact harmless. We can expose ourselves to spiders to lessen spider phobia. But we cannot send military veterans with PTSD back to the front for therapeutic purposes, because war is not harmless. The woman cannot seek repeated traumatic sex so as to desensitize herself to being abused. That said, no less, the Dutch Royal Science Society (Koninklijke Nederlandse Academie van Wetenschappen; KNAW, 2011) wrote in the national science agenda: 'If a child is a possible victim of sexual abuse, we could expose her to pictures of abuse situations and register the child's brain activity' (p. 76). That sounds like a strange idea to me, to say the least. One final challenge for the primary hypothesis in this case is that dissociative complaints are intrusive. That implies that they cannot be consciously controlled. Hence, it is virtually impossible that the woman would have been able to deliberately get into a dissociative trance whenever she had sex with her social worker.

6.2 The Verdict

Based on the report by Dr. Israels and me, the court decided that it was not certain that the woman was indeed subconscious during the sexual encounters. Therefore, the suspect was acquitted from rape. He was convicted nonetheless for having sex with someone who was subjected to his care. Even though he was off the woman's case professionally, and she knew that, the court still believed that in her eyes the social worker was someone whom she could trust to serve her best interest. His penalty was 3 days of imprisonment and 240 h of public service.

References

American Psychiatric Association (APA). (2013). *Diagnostic and statistical manual of mental disorders* (5th ed.). APA.

Brewin, C. R., & Mersaditabari, N. (2013). Experimentally-induced dissociation impairs visual memory. *Consciousness & Cognition, 22*, 1189–1194.

Eysenck, H. J. (1994). The outcome problem in psychotherapy: What have we learned? *Behaviour Research and Therapy, 32*, 477–495.

Gershuny, B. S., & Thayer, J. F. (1999). Relations among psychological trauma, dissociative phenomena, and trauma-related distress: A review and integration. *Clinical Psychology Review, 19*, 631–657.

Huntjens, R. J. C., Peters, M. L., Woertman, L., van der Hart, O., & Postma, A. (2007). Memory transfer for emotionally valenced words between identities in dissociative identity disorder. *Behaviour Research and Therapy, 45*, 775–789.

Kindt, M., & van den Hout, M. (2003). Dissociation and memory fragmentation: Experimental effects on meta-memory but not on actual memory performance. *Behaviour Research and Therapy, 41*, 167–178.

Koninklijke Nederlandse Academie van Wetenschappen (KNAW). (2011). *De Nederlandse wetenschapsagenda*. KNAW.

Mangiulli, I., Otgaar, H., Jelicic, M., & Merckelbach, H. (2022). A critical review of case studies on dissociative amnesia. *Clinical Psychological Science, 10*(2), 191–211.

Merckelbach, H., & Patihis, L. (2018). Why "trauma-related dissociation" is a misnomer in courts: A critical analysis of brand et al. (2017a, b). *Psychological Inquiry and Law, 11*, 370–376.

Otgaar, H., Howe, M. L., Patihis, L., Merckelbach, H., Lynn, S. J., Lilienfeld, S. O., & Loftus, E. F. (2019). The return of the repressed: The persistent and problematic claims of long-forgotten trauma. *Perspectives on Psychological Science, 14*(6), 1072–1095.

Chapter 7
The Tantra Therapist and the Threat of Collaborative Storytelling

In 2017, six women filed complaints against a 52-year-old man. They accused him of sexual misconduct and rape. He admitted that he had had intimate contact with all these women, but strictly within the context of Tantra therapy. In this therapy, intimate contact is a means of breaking personal blockades that hinder happiness. The women knew that intimate touching was involved, but they claimed that the therapist had gone too far, further than they had agreed, and/or wanted him to go. Nonetheless, all women had taken multiple therapy sessions with the suspect between 2013 and 2017. The suspect's defence asked for an opinion on the veracity of the six allegations. The defence found it problematic that the women had discussed with each other their experiences with the therapist often before they decided to go to the police.

In my report, I discussed the alternative scenario in which the women spoke about their experiences and thus influenced each other's recollection and testimonies. I referred to Crombag (1999) who described a case that somewhat resembles the present one. In that case, an artist, Edward Green, had sexual relations with several of his nude models. Ultimately, four of these models made accusations of sexual assault. According to the author, these accusations were the result of prolonged discussion between these four women. Initially, they did not know each other. Once they got to know each other (they were all art students), and learned of their shared intimacy with the artist, they must have been slightly confused. Hence, they discussed their experience intensively. During these discussions, they must have discovered that their sexual behaviour was not typical of them. Concluding that the artist had actually abused them, made their own sexual behaviour seem less active and voluntary, and made them feel less bad about themselves. Thus, this changed interpretation was a means to reduce cognitive dissonance. Crombag called this process collaborative storytelling. He emphasises that this is not a manifestation of lying. The discussions actually altered the women's recollection of what had happened during their sexual encounters.

ECLI:NL:RBMNE:2019:1709

E. Rassin, *Case Studies in Legal Psychology*,
https://doi.org/10.1007/978-3-031-44931-4_7

Arguably, the changed emotional evaluation of the sexual experiences is a slight reconstruction of memory, at least compared to most of the literature on false memories discussed in Chap. 6. That is, it has been shown repeatedly that we easily fall prey to false memories. The concept of collaborative storytelling does not actually require a false memory but merely a change in the evaluation of the experienced event. Such a change is the primary purpose of EMDR, albeit in that therapy the change is in the positive direction, whereas in collaborative storytelling it is in the opposite direction. That said, there is little research directly addressing the effects of collaborative storytelling. One relevant study was done by Tversky and Marsh (2000). In one of their experiments, these authors had participants read a story about a murder. There were two suspects, and hence, some information was incriminating to one of the suspects, while other information was incriminating for the other. Finally, there was ambiguous information. Part of the participants were instructed to write down all they could remember from the murder case. The other half were instructed to write as if their writing was to convince a jury that one of the suspects had to be convicted. Later, all participants underwent a free recall test. It turned out that those who had written a selective reproduction previously (i.e., the story that had to convince the jury) had now actually a worse recollection of the story than those who had written a neutral reproduction. Apparently, writing a selective argumentative reproduction had, possibly due to selective rehearsal, actually resulted in decreased, selective memory. Note that in this instance, there was only little suggestion. The only suggestive intervention was the instruction to write a juicy version of the original event, which resulted in an actual alteration of memory in the later neutral recall test.

Hope et al. (2008) showed a one-and-a-half-minute film clip about a woman entering a room to 96 undergraduates. However, the woman was simultaneously filmed from two different angles, and thus there were two versions of the film. Only in one version the woman could be seen steeling ten pounds. Sometime later, participants answered questions about the film. In the meantime, some participants had discussed the film with one other person. The study was designed so that the other person always had seen the other version of the film. Further, the relation between the two participants differed. They were either strangers, friends, or couples. During free recall, none of the participants in the no-discussion condition, who had seen the film without the theft, reported that the woman took money. However, of those who had discussed the film with a stranger, 17% did report to have seen her steel money. In the friends and couples conditions, this percentage was 50%. Further, on average 54% of participants who had not seen the theft confirmed that they did when asked the (leading) question of whether they believed that the girl was guilty of theft.

Another study with relevance to the present case is by Kaasa et al. (2013) who had 129 undergraduates participate in a (bogus) study in which their height, weight, blood pressure, and other measures were taken by a female lab assistant. One month later, each participant received a phone call in which they were asked how the lab assistant had behaved. The participants told the interviewer that the assistant had behaved normally, which was true, because she was part of the research team and behaved neatly on each occasion. However, the interviewer would then say: ‘Are you sure she didn't say anything inappropriate? I know this happened a few weeks ago, so why don't you think about it for a minute?'. The interviewer asked the participants whether they were willing to sign a complaint form about the lab assistant that had already been signed by a number of participants. This complaint form was to be used to build a case against the assistant, and would be anonymous. Two weeks later, participants were called again and were again asked whether they would sign a complaint form, but some of them were told that their names would appear on the form. In the first interview, no less than 38.8% of the participants were willing to sign the complaint. In the second interview, 14.8% of the participants were willing to sign the form. These findings illustrate that people are quite easily brought to utter false allegations when asked so. When debriefed and asked why they had signed the complaint, most participants (38.8%) reported to have been willing to do so to help other participants. Some of them (12.2%) did so because they did not like the lab assistant.

As said, none of these experiments specifically addressed the core of collaborative storytelling, namely that the emotional evaluation of an experienced event can change due to discussion with others. Nonetheless, the findings reiterate that such a change is far from imaginary or impossible. Notably, the present case did in many respects resemble the one described by Crombag (1999). For one thing, the six victims knew beforehand that sexual touching was a possibility in the Tantra sessions. Some of them admitted that that was exactly what they were looking for. The verdict contains many quotes from the victims. Some of these are: 'Our intimate sessions were meant to bring me more in touch with my feelings. The sex was aimed at dearmouring', 'There was coaching in the form of touching and being touched, and "I wanted a Tantra massage, being touched all over my body'. One client even produced a written agreement stating that she would be touched sexually during the sessions. While some women claimed that the therapist went too far, or further than was agreed beforehand, they all knew that there was a grey area of intimate touching. None of them experienced the sex as unwanted, and they all went back for more.

The case also resembles the one described by Crombag (1999) in that the women self-reported to have developed feelings that were not necessary for their treatment per se. Here are some examples of quotes that hint in that direction: 'I had developed feelings for him … I told him I loved him … I felt flattered because he made me feel special', 'I got addicted to him … I fell in love with him', 'I got dependent because I found him extremely cute. I wanted to keep him. I was scared of losing him', 'I felt special. He said that I was the only one to whom he did these things. I was vulnerable'. Finally, these arguably positive feelings turned sour when the women got into contact (through social media) and started discussing their experiences. Notable, the extensive discussions between the women, preceding the allegations, were not disputed and even well-documented.

The court accepted the possibility of collaborative storytelling in that the judges left open that the women 'may not have experienced the sexual encounters as unwanted at the time'. The suspect was convicted nonetheless based on a different legal argumentation. That is, the court established that the suspect and the women had sex in the context of a therapeutic relationship. And sex between a therapist and a client is by definition prohibited, according to the Dutch Supreme Court's jurisprudence. The only exception is if the sex occurs fully outside of the ongoing therapeutic relationship. The suspect was convicted to 30 months of imprisonment, between roughly 2500 and 7000 euro damages to the six victims, and a prohibition to act as Tantra therapist for 4 years. In court, he had already testified that he considered stopping Tantra therapy.

References

Crombag, H. F. M. (1999). Collaborative story-telling: A hypothesis in need of experimental testing. *Psychology, Crime & Law, 5*, 279–289.

Hope, L., Ost, J., Gabbert, F., Healy, S., & Lenton, E. (2008). "With a little help from my friends …": The role of co-witness relationship in susceptibility to misinformation. *Acta Psychologica, 127*, 467–484.

Kaasa, S. O., Cauffman, E., Clarke-Stewart, K. A., & Loftus, E. F. (2013). False accusations in an investigative context: Differences between suggestible and non-suggestible witnesses. *Behavioral Sciences & the Law, 31*, 574–592.

Tversky, B., & Marsh, E. J. (2000). Biased retellings of events yield biased memories. *Cognitive Psychology, 40*, 1–38.

Chapter 8
Magic Mumfry and the Snowball Effect

In 2015, a 30-year-old swim instructor was brought to trial, because of suspicion of sexually maltreating 26 pupils. Allegedly, he touched these children in their genital zone during the swim lessons. Among the alleged victims were both boys and girls. Of course, the children did not disclose their experiences simultaneously. It started with one boy who made a remark about being pinched in the bottom during swim lesson to his mother. In the months that followed, more children disclosed the maltreatment, and their parents and caretakers eventually filed allegation on behalf of them. The suspect denied. That is, he testified that the swim lessons require the instructor to touch the children often to correct their posture, but these touches were purely functional. Inappropriate touches, if any, were accidental. The defence asked me for an opinion on the 26 allegations.

8.1 The Effect of Rumours

Intuitively, the evidence for the primary hypothesis is strong in this case, if for no other reason, because the number of allegations is impressively high. Where there is smoke, there is fire. It seems implausible that so many children would be mistaken. Admittedly though, the 26 eventual cases stem from a much larger pool of potential victims, because the suspect had taught hundreds of children how to swim.

Under the alternative hypothesis, the initial boy's allegations were based on a mistaken interpretation of a functional touch, and most of the subsequent allegations were merely due to children copycatting. There were indications that all children had talked about the suspect and the allegations. There is some research suggesting that children do indeed copycat readily. This copycatting may affect memory. Children's memory is in some respects different from memory in

ECLI:RBNHO:2015:2530

E. Rassin, *Case Studies in Legal Psychology*,
https://doi.org/10.1007/978-3-031-44931-4_8

adulthood. One peculiarity of children's memory is infantile or childhood amnesia, which refers to a general inability to recall events in the first years of our life. Multhaup et al. (2005) adopted an interesting approach to find out to which age childhood amnesia extends. They gave undergraduates a list with common events, and asked whether the students merely knew that they had experienced the event, or had actual memories of the event. Some events generally occur earlier (e.g., one's first word, first time standing, walking) than others (e.g., swimming lessons, visit to movie theatre, sleepover, biking). Based on the know-recollect distinction, the authors computed that for adults, childhood amnesia extends to the first 4.5 years of our lives.

In some respects, children's memory may be superior to that of adults. For instance, Brainerd et al. (2008) studied 17 publications, describing 26 experiments employing the previously discussed DRM paradigm (see Roediger & McDermott, 1995) in various age groups ranging from three through the early twenties. They concluded that the false recall of critical lures increases with age. It even roughly triples between the age of five and early adolescence. False recognition roughly doubles during this time span. The authors speak of developmental reversals, referring to a paradoxical decrease of specific memory performance with age. This particular reversal is probably due to children not making the association between the presented words, which prevents them from internally generating associated lures.

Despite the specific developmental reversals, there is much research on children's suggestibility and consequent apparent memory distortion. Obviously, the topic of false memories of unpleasant experiences is sensitive and difficult research wise. While research on false allegations is thus challenging, there is some research suggesting that children are indeed susceptible to suggestion by adults and also to peer pressure, which may ultimately result in false incriminating testimonies. Principe et al. (2006) took 175 pre-schoolers to Magic Mumfry's show, to witness Mumfry failing to pull the rabbit out of his hat as his final trick. Soon afterwards, some of the children witnessed the rabbit walking through the school. Others did not, but overheard a conversation between two adults, in which it was mentioned that the rabbit had escaped and walked through the school, and hence the trick failed. Yet another part of the children merely were classmates of the children who overheard the conversation. Finally, a subsample of children underwent none of the interventions after the magic show. The findings yielded 100% true positives (i.e., all of the children who had actually seen the rabbit reported to have seen it) after 1 week. Meanwhile, 38% of the children who had overheard the conversation claimed to have seen the rabbit, and 68% of their classmates did to. of the children in the control condition claimed to have None seen the rabbit. Notably, some of the children had been exposed to suggestive interviews prior to the final interview. For those children, 70% in the overhear condition, 78% in the classmate condition, and even 23% in the control condition claimed to have witnessed the rabbit walking loose in the school. Principe et al. (2007) tested whether false accusations also occur if the overheard rumour about the loose walking rabbit is at odds with children's own experience. One hundred and thirty two pre-schoolers witnessed Mumfry's failed attempt to pull the rabbit out of the hat. Half of them subsequently saw that

Mumfry went searching for the rabbit and found it in its cage. According to Mumfry, the rabbit was sick, and therefore disliked leaving his cage. He gave the rabbit some medicine. Later, some children overheard the adult conversation about the rabbit having escaped and walking loose through the school. Hence, for some of them, this rumour was at odds with what they had just witnessed. In the interview, 1 week later, 42% of the 3–4-year-olds who had overheard the rumour (but had not seen Mumfry give the rabbit medicine) falsely claimed to have seen the rabbit walking through the school, but so did 58% of those whose experience was at odds with the rumour. Corresponding percentages for the 5–6 year olds were 33% in the non-conflicting, and 9% in the conflicting condition. Hence, especially in the younger sample, false accusations were not tempered by conflicting experience. Principe et al. (2010) slightly adapted the magic Mumfry paradigm so as to test whether peer influence is crucial for the spreading of the rumour. After overhearing the conversation, some children were allowed 30 minutes of free play, whereas others spent 30 minutes without free play. After 1 week, 38% of the children in the former condition claimed to have seen the rabbit walking loose, while 11% of those in the latter condition did so. By and large, this finding supports the hypothesis that peer influence is detrimental for the accuracy of narratives. In their second study, all 57 children were granted 30 min of play time. However, half of the children were classmates, whereas in the unfamiliar condition, the children did not know each other. False claims of seeing the rabbit occurred in 41% in the former, and 7% in the latter condition, again supporting the effect of social influence. Finally, Principe et al. (2012) replicated the findings in a sample of 123 pre-schoolers. Some children overheard the adult conversation, while others were merely their classmates. In this experiment, children were interviewed twice, after 1 and 4 weeks. In the younger groups (aged 3–4 years), 44% of the children in the overhear condition and 75% in the classmate condition claimed having seen the rabbit, after 1 week. Three weeks later, the corresponding percentages were 39% and 75%. In the older samples (aged 5–6), 14% of the children who had overheard the conversation and 35% of their classmates claimed to have seen the rabbit, after 1 week. After 4 weeks, 10% in the former and 35% in the latter condition did so.

Some of the main findings in the studies by Principe and colleagues are summarized in Table 8.1 (see also Principe & Schindewolf, 2012, for a review). The percentages are weighted if the information in the articles allowed so. In the bottom row, an overall, partly weighted mean is presented. It can be concluded that children are quite susceptible to suggestion by adults but also, and possibly even more so by peer pressure. It must further be acknowledged that in absence of suggestion, the children did quite well, both in terms of sensitivity and specificity.

In all, these findings suggest that once there is an initial allegation or even a rumour that the swim instructor pinched one of the children under water, and children discuss this and are asked about it by their parents, there is a considerable likelihood of around 36% that those who have no experience still would fiercely claim that they were pinched as well. Arguably then, under the alternative hypothesis, if the rumour was spread among 75 children or more, it would be possible that 26 false positive allegations came about.

Table 8.1 Main findings in the studies by Principe and colleagues

	True positive likelihood	Completely spontaneous false positive likelihood	False positive likelihood after any kind of suggestion
Principe and Ceci (2002)	78%	0%	36%
Principe et al. (2006)	100%	0%	56%
Principe et al. (2007)	–	12%	35%
Principe et al. (2010)	–	0%	22%
Principe et al. (2012)	–	0%	29%
Overall	89%	2.4%	36%

As to the ending of this case, the court wrote in the verdict that they were aware of the risk of mutual influencing between the children, and of the leading questions asked by the parents. Nonetheless, the court found the testimonies authentic, spontaneous, and trustworthy. In addition, because there were so many allegations, they served as support for each other. The suspect was convicted to 3 years in prison, and approximately 1000 euro damages to be paid to many of the 26 victims.

References

Brainerd, C. J., Reyna, V. F., & Ceci, S. J. (2008). Developmental reversals in false memory: A review of data and theory. *Psychological Bulletin, 134*, 343–382.

Multhaup, K. S., Johnson, M. D., & Tetirick, J. C. (2005). The wane of childhood amnesia for autobiographical and public event memories. *Memory, 13*, 161–173.

Principe, G. F., & Ceci, S. J. (2002). "I saw it with my own ears": The effects of peer conversations on preschoolers' reports of nonexperienced events. *Journal of Experimental Child Psychology, 83*, 1–25.

Principe, G. F., & Schindewolf, E. (2012). Natural conversations as a source of false memories in children: Implications for the testimony of young witnesses. *Developmental Review, 32*, 205–223.

Principe, G. F., Kanaya, T., Ceci, S. J., & Singh, M. (2006). Believing is seeing: How rumors can engender false memories in preschoolers. *Psychological Science, 17*, 243–248.

Principe, G. F., Tinguely, A., & Dobkowski, N. (2007). Mixing memories: The effects of rumors that conflict with children's experiences. *Journal of Experimental Child Psychology, 98*, 1–19.

Principe, G. F., Daley, L., & Kauth, K. (2010). Social processes affecting the mnemonic consequences of rumors on children's memory. *Journal of Experimental Child Psychology, 107*, 479–493.

Principe, G. F., Cherson, M., DiPuppo, J., & Schindewolf, E. (2012). Children's natural conversations following exposure to a rumor: Linkage to later false reports. *Journal of Experimental Child Psychology, 113*, 383–400.

Roediger, H. L., & McDermott, K. B. (1995). Creating false memories: Remembering words not presented in lists. *Journal of Experimental Psychology: Learning, Memory and Cognition, 24*, 803–814.

Chapter 9
A Shocked and Caring Community

In 2011, a 53-year-old man was charged with alleged sexual abuse of three young girls. He was suspected of having touched the children inappropriately during swim lessons he gave them. The abuse was considered to have taken place in 2010. He was also suspected of having abused his stepdaughter (now 31 years) when she was approximately 5 years old. This abuse was thus in the distant past. Finally, during the search of the suspect's home, the police found a forbidden rifle. The suspect denied the abuse. Inappropriate touches of the three girls, if any, were unintended and functional. An independent witness testified that she had seen the suspect benignly helping one of the girls with adjusting her suit after returning from the toilet. It was possible that this instance was at the root of this girl's allegation. The abuse of the stepdaughter was denied categorically by the suspect. As to the gun, the suspect testified that he had owned it for a long time and did not wish to part from it, even though he knew it was forbidden. The court asked for an opinion on the allegations of the four alleged victims.

9.1 The Information Session

The first disclosure was made by the girl who was helped adjusting her swimsuit (according to the suspect and a third person). The girl testified that during this incident, the suspect had touched her bottom. The girl's parents went to the management of the swimming pool. The management suspended the suspect from work. Of course, the possibility of abuse was shocking to the parents and caregivers of the children who took swim lessons in this pool. Assuming that the rumour would spread anyway, and to prevent troubles, stress, and confusion, one evening, the management of the swimming pool organised, together with city hall officials and the

---

ECLI:NL:RBAMS:2012:BV1244

E. Rassin, *Case Studies in Legal Psychology*,
https://doi.org/10.1007/978-3-031-44931-4_9

prosecution's office, an information session for all parents whose children had taken lessons from the suspect. During the information evening, the suspect's first name plus initial of his surname were mentioned. His defence found that careless, albeit that even if this had not been mentioned, most people involved would still have been able to figure out who the suspect was. Further, no less than 2000 people were invited to the information session, of which many were not parents or caregivers of children who had taken swim lessons from the suspect.

Subsequent to the information evening, four allegations were made to the police. First, there was the girl who claimed to have been touched when her swimsuit was straightened. Two girls alleged that the suspect had touched their butts when they swam on their back. The suspect's stepdaughter testified that the suspect had once penetrated her anally with a thermometer. The suspect later testified that he may well have done so because they used to take temperature rectally. However, the stepdaughter claimed that she referred to a toy thermometer, and that the penetration was purely sexual.

From a legal psychological stance, the alternative hypothesis in this case is that the suspect had not touched any of the victims sexually, but purely functionally, and that the three girls came to their allegations because of unintended coaching by their parents. Understandably, parents who fear that their child may have been touched inappropriately will have their child's best interest at heart, less so the possibility that their questions may falsely implicate the swim instructor (Korkman et al., 2014). There is some research suggesting that children are quite susceptible to leading questions posed by adults. A classic study is the Sam Stone experiment by Leichtman and Ceci (1995). These authors included 176 pre-schoolers (aged 3 through 6 years) in their study. All children were visited by a stranger, named Sam Stone, in their classroom. The encounter lasted for about 2 min during which Sam walked through the room, told the children that the story they were being read by the teacher was his favourite, and left. Ten weeks later, the children were interviewed about Sam's visit. During this interview, an open question was asked ('Remember the day Sam Stone visited the school? Well, I wasn't there that day, and I'd like you to tell me everything that happened when he visited'). Later on, a probe question was asked ('Have you heard something about a book or teddy bear?'). If this probe was affirmed, the child was asked whether he had actually seen this. Finally, if the child indicated he had indeed witnessed the pertinent event, a critical question was asked ('You didn't really see him do this, did you?'). As described so far, the procedure matched the control condition. However, there were three experimental conditions. In the stereotype condition, children were coached four times, spread over a month before Sam's visit by a confederate who described Sam as a kind friend who is clumsy and regularly breaks things accidentally. In the suggestion condition, children were interviewed four times after Sam's visit, yet before the final interview after 10 weeks. During these four interviews, suggestive remarks were made about Sam's visit, particularly that he had destroyed a book and soiled a teddy bear. Finally, children in the combined stereotype and suggestion condition received suggestions prior and posterior to Sam's visit. With this design, Leichtman and Ceci could register what the effects of coaching and suggestion were on the

Table 9.1 Percentages of false accusation as a function of pre-interview coaching and suggestion (Leichtman & Ceci, 1995)

Condition	Question during final interview	Percentage of children falsely accusing Sam		
		3–4 years	5–6 years	Overall
Control	Open	0	0	0
	Probe	10	3.5	6.2
	Witnessed?	5	0	2
	Critical	2.5	0	1
Stereotype	Open	0	0	0
	Probe	37	19	27
	Witnessed?	18	9	13
	Critical	10	2.5	7.4
Suggestion	Open	21	14	17.6
	Probe	53	38	45.1
	Witnessed?	35	10	22
	Critical	12	9.1	9.3
Stereotype + suggestion	Open	46	30	38.5
	Probe	72	38	57.7
	Witnessed?	44	14	31.8
	Critical	21	5	14.4

neutral interview after 10 weeks. Findings are summarised in Table 9.1. Ignoring age effects, and assuming that in a correct interview, there is some probing, and also some critical questioning (in my personal experience, interviews indeed include some probing, but hardly or no critical questions), children were unlikely to spontaneously include false accusations in their testimonies (i.e., 1%). If coached, the likelihood increased to 7.4% to 9.3% after suggestive pre-interview discussion, and even to 14.4% after both coaching and suggestion.

In a conceptual replication, Principe and Ceci (2002) had 96 pre-schoolers participate in an archaeology session led by Dr. Diggs. Four weeks later, they were interviewed about this event. Some participants underwent three suggestive interviews prior to the final interview. In these interviews, the children were exposed to suggestive questions about Dr. Diggs smearing a precious treasure map and breaking a rock. However, some children were allocated to the witness condition, in which they actually saw Dr. Diggs ruin the two valuable items. During the final interview, open, specific, source, and countersuggestion questions were asked. Findings suggested that only 34% of the children in the witness condition spontaneously mentioned that Dr. Diggs had ruined the two artefacts. The percentage of true positives increased to 81% after specific questions, remained 78% when asked if actually witnessed, and dropped to 44% after the countersuggestion ('You didn't really see him do that, did you?'). As to the false positives, approximately 37% of the children spontaneously mentioned the accusations, 72% did so after specific questions, 44% maintained to have seen the acts, and 25% kept up after the critical intervention.

In a study by Principe et al. (2013) in which the effect of discussion between the children and their mother was tested, 117 pre-schoolers attended Mumfry's magic show ending with the failed rabbit trick. One week later, they were interviewed about the show. One day before the interview, some children received a letter to be handed over to their mother. In this letter, the mothers were invited to ask their child about the show in a neutral manner (e.g., 'Tell me what happened during the magic show at your school'). Part of the children received a version of the letter in which was added that the mother should ask if the child 'remembers whether the magician's rabbit got loose in the school'. In this instance, the researchers did not inquire whether the children claimed seeing the rabbit themselves. Nonetheless, 8% of the children in the neutral letter condition mentioned that the rabbit had escaped, while 60% of the children whose mother had read a suggestive letter did so.

A study by Otgaar et al. (2008) deserves some attention because it addressed to what extent false memories of bizarre events can occur in children. The authors were interested in three variables: Age, content of the false memory, and presence of additional information supporting the occurrence of the target event. There were 44 children aged 7–8 years and 47 aged 11–12 years. Some of the children were told that they had been abducted by a UFO when they were 4 years old (bizarre event). Others were told that they had almost choked on a candy. Finally, some children were shown a fake newspaper report about alleged alien abductions to support the (false) memory. In the young age group, 45% of the children reported to remember almost having choked when presented with prevalence information about choking, while 40% did so in absence of prevalence information. The authors succeeded to implant false memories of an alien abduction in 21% of the younger children without supporting prevalence information, and in no less than 78% if combined with prevalence information. In the older age group, false memories occurred less often, bizarre events were falsely remembered less often, and prevalence information did not fuel false memories. That is, 23% of the children believed to have choked without, and 45% with prevalence information. As to the bizarre event, 8% of the older children developed false memories in presence and 18% in absence of prevalence information. A second interview, 1 week later, yielded similar results. By and large, the findings suggest that the elicitation of false narratives is not limited to insignificant events, but stretches out to bizarre, unbelievable, or even unimaginable ones too.

In all, research findings such as those discussed here suggest that children are not only susceptible to peer pressure as discussed in Chap. 8, but also to informal coaching by adults.

9.2 Anatomically Detailed Drawings

There was another aspect in this case that was addressed in my forensic report. That is, some of the interventions in the interview of the three girls were quite suggestive and that may have contributed to false allegations (under the alternative hypothesis). This was so in the interview of two of the girls because they only came up with incriminating details after and in response to the suggestions. Even though police interviews can generally be expected to be bias-free, it cannot be excluded that an interviewer accidentally poses a crucial leading question. To check the quality (i.e., the absence of suggestion) of the interview, it has to be literally transcribed in a so-called verbatim report. Even better is that the audio(−visual) registration of the interview is made available to the legal psychologist. The latter was the case in this instance. Several suggestive interventions might occur in a police interview, some of which are more subtle than others. For example, in child interviews, (repeated) closed questions might work coercively (Andrews & Lamb, 2014; Pichler et al., 2021). Likewise, an encouraging remark (e.g., 'Come on, you must know that') and selectively reinforcing incriminating remarks are considered to be coercive. Obviously, a (child-)witness who does not know the answer to a question should not be encouraged to speculate or imagine what the answer might be. The interviewer should give a proper instruction at the onset of the interview, including that the (child-)witness is free to talk in his own words, that he should admit if he does not remember the answer to a question, that the witness should correct the interviewer if a mistake is made, and that the witness should mention if something is unclear. Further, it is important that the interviewer remains empathic but detached, and not be tempted to take up the role of therapist. This might be difficult if the (child-)witness is very emotional. The interviewer should remain distant enough to make non-accusing critical remarks, for example, if there are crucial inconsistencies in the testimony. Such critical remarks are important to test alternative scenarios. If multiple witnesses have to be interviewed, it is recommendable that each witness is interviewed by a different interviewer, to avoid cross-over effects and interviewer bias. A subtle mistake, of interest to the legal psychologist, is that the child-witness is interviewed in the presence of a parent. It might seem good that the child is supported by a parent during the interview. It may even make it easier to talk about the alleged crime. However, all this is only so in the primary scenario. But in an alternative scenario in which the child is coached by the parent to make false allegation, allowing the parent to be present during the interview suppresses the already small likelihood that the child will admit that the parent coached him into giving false testimony.

A final example of a subtle leading intervention is the use of anatomically detailed dolls or drawings (ADDs; see Fig. 9.1). These props are used in child interviews to clarify witness statements. However, research suggests that ADDs may elicit false allegations. Willcock et al. (2006) took 125 5–6-year-olds to the fire station where they were assisted to take on a fire suit. While putting on the suit, a confederate fireman touched the children in five places including their armpits. One month later, the children were interviewed about their visit to the fire station. During this interview, a dressed ADD was presented to the children so as to mark the places where the fireman had touched them. On average, the children marked only 37.6% of the places they had been touched. Children also marked 3.6 places in which they had actually not been touched. Consequently, less than half (47.8%) of the marked places in the ADD were accurate. Crucially, 11.3% of the children marked the genital zone in the ADD (see also Poole et al., 2011).

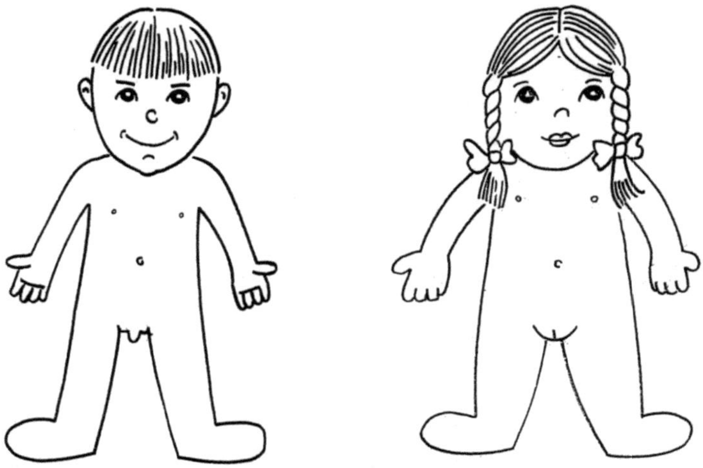

Fig. 9.1 Anatomically detailed drawings

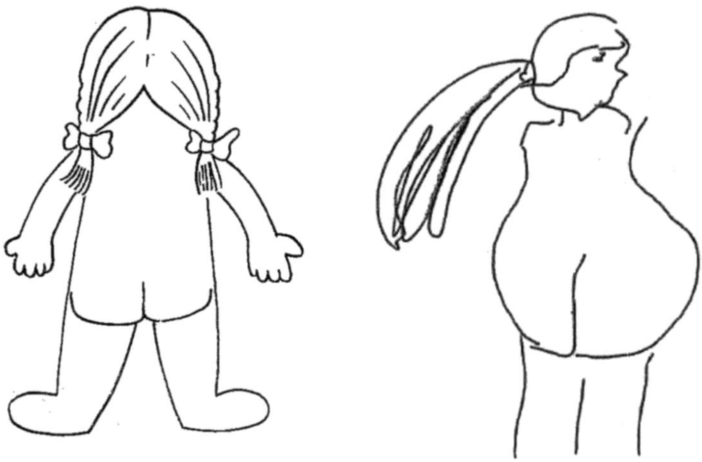

Fig. 9.2 Standard ADD of female back (left), and the one created in this case (right)

In one of the interviews, the interviewer sought to show an ADD to the girl. However, there was no ADD present in the interview room. ADDs had recently been banned from use, because of critique by legal psychologists based on the research discussed above. Possibly, the interviewer was unaware of this new policy. He had conducted the interview with one of the other girls who had told him that the suspect touched her behind while she was swimming on her back, and he wanted to ask the current interviewee whether she was also touched in the same place, even before the child had mentioned any of this to him spontaneously. When he could not find an ADD like the one in the left panel of Fig. 9.2, he ad hoc made his own version which looked like the one in the right panel of Fig. 9.2. I commented negatively on the use of drawings in general, and particularly on the version created in this interview because of the disproportionately big behind.

A few years after this case, Dodier and Denault (2018) introduced the Griffiths questionograph with which the quality of an interview can be summarised graphically. They distinguish no less than nine types of verbal interventions, but still this tool cannot capture all possible suggestions. In their classification, three question types are appropriate: Open questions, probing questions ('what', 'where', 'who', 'when', 'how'), and closed questions (concluding a topic). Six question types are inappropriate: Open questions that interrupt the free recall, inappropriate closed questions (e.g., 'Do you know this man?'), multiple questions, forced choice questions, opinions, and leading questions ('Are you usually that aggressive when drunk?'). The authors number these nine types of questions in a way that appropriate questions are given higher scores (7–9), and inappropriate ones receive lower scores (1–6). The example in Fig. 9.3, then, represents an interview fragment that starts with an open question, and a follow-up open question that interrupts the witness. In all, this interview fragment appears to be of low quality, because only 5 of the 15 questions are appropriate. Hence, the questionograph offers a neat and quick overview of the quality of an interview (fragment). This is not only handy for teaching purposes, but also for the evaluation of the alternative scenario in which the incriminating evidence included in a testimony can be attributed to suggestion during the interview. It is important to note that the effect of a coercive intervention is likely to be stronger at the beginning of the interview than later on. In fact, a coercive intervention is only detrimental if the witness is actually affected by the intervention. If this happens at the beginning of the interview, all information subsequently provided by the witness about the pertinent topic may be invalid.

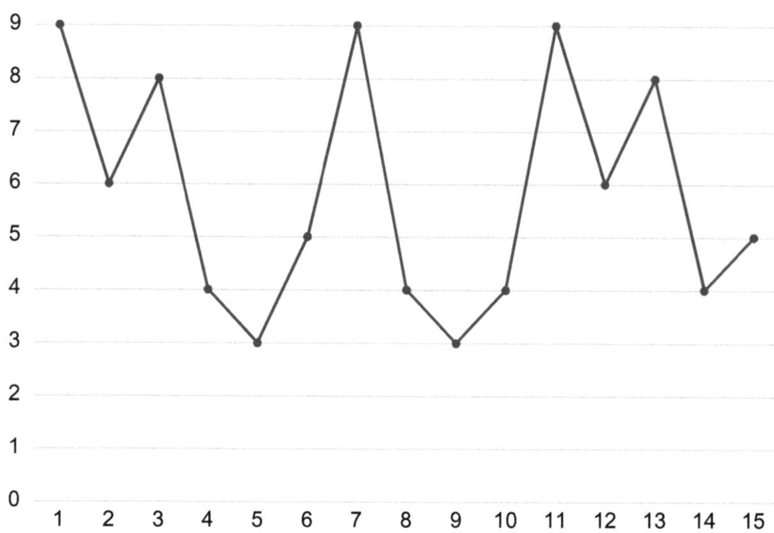

Fig. 9.3 Fictitious example of a Griffiths questionograph

9.3 How This Case Ended

In my report, I stressed the potential alternative hypothesis of a false allegation caused by a misinterpretation of the suspect's attempt to adjust girl 1's swimsuit, suggestion fuelled by the public information session, and subsequently by the parents of girls 2 and 3, poor quality of the police interview (particularly in girl 3's case where the self-drawn backside was used), and reconstructive memory affected by psychotherapy in case of the suspect's stepdaughter.

The defence argued that the testimonies of the three girls should be declared inadmissible, because the prosecution had acted carelessly in programming the information session, and the police had conducted poor quality interviews.

The court did not go as far as the defence requested, but did acquit the suspect from most charges. As to girl 1, the judges decided that her testimony was authentic, but the touches were not sexual but purely functional in adjusting the girl's suit. The testimonies of girls 2 and 3 had suppressed evidentiary power because of the poor quality of their interviews. Hence, the suspect was acquitted of these allegations. He was also acquitted of the allegations brought forward by the stepdaughter, because there was no evidence corroborating her claims. The suspect was convicted of illegal possession of firearms. He was sentenced to 1 month imprisonment with subtraction of the time spent in arrest (which had been more than 1 month).

The prosecution disagreed and went on appeal. The appeal court maintained the acquittal of allegations made by girls 2 and 3. However, the judges did convict the suspect for sexual misconduct towards the first girl, because they refused to assume that the suspect had purely functional intent. They also found him guilty of abusing his stepdaughter, because she had previously disclosed allegations around 2003. In all, he was sentenced to 18 months of imprisonment.

References

Andrews, S. J., & Lamb, M. E. (2014). The effects of age and delay on responses to repeated questions in forensic interviews with children alleging sexual abuse. *Law and Human Behavior, 38*(2), 171–180.

Dodier, O., & Denault, V. (2018). The Griffiths question map: A forensic tool for expert witnesses' assessments of witnesses and victims' statements. *Journal of Forensic Sciences, 63*, 266–274.

Korkman, J., Juusola, A., & Santtila, P. (2014). Who made the disclosure? Recorded discussions between children and caretakers suspecting child abuse. *Psychology, Crime & Law, 20*, 994–1004.

Leichtman, M. D., & Ceci, S. J. (1995). The effects of stereotypes and suggestions on preschoolers' reports. *Developmental Psychology, 31*, 568–578.

Otgaar, H., Candel, I., Merckelbach, H., & Wade, K. A. (2008). Abducted by a UFO: Prevalence information affects children's false memories for an implausible event. *Applied Cognitive Psychology, 23*, 115–125.

Pichler, A. S., Powell, M., Sharman, S. J., Zyderveldt, S., Westera, N., & Goodman-Delanhunty, J. (2021). Inconsistencies in complainant's accounts of child sexual abuse arising in their cross-examination. *Psychology Crime and Law, 27*(4), 341–356.

Poole, D. A., Bruck, M., & Pipe, M. E. (2011). Forensic interviewing aids: Do props help children answer questions about touching? *Current Directions in Psychological Science, 20*, 11–15.

Principe, G. F., & Ceci, S. J. (2002). "I saw it with my own ears": The effects of peer conversations on preschoolers' reports of nonexperienced events. *Journal of Experimental Child Psychology, 83*, 1–25.

Principe, G. F., DiPuppo, J., & Gammel, J. (2013). Effects of mothers' conversation style and receipt of misinformation on children's event reports. *Cognitive Development, 28*, 260–271.

Willcock, E., Morgan, K., & Hayne, H. (2006). Body maps do not facilitate children's reports of touch. *Applied Cognitive Psychology, 20*, 607–615.

Chapter 10
The Amnestic Murderer

In the afternoon of March 10, 2013, the police get a phone call in which they are informed about a capital crime. Upon arrival at the crime scene, they find a 54-year-old male suspect, the dead body of his wife, and the suspect's brother who had arrived at the suspect's home earlier and had called the police. According to the policeman who talked to the suspect first, he said 'I did it, it is my fault'. Apparently, the suspect had strangled his wife. There was also much blood at the crime scene, but that was the suspect's own. The suspect maintained his confession during various interviews for 3 months. He testified that he was very depressed, particularly since he lost his job. Eventually, he wanted to commit suicide. The fact that he gave care to his sick wife had long time prevented him from carrying out his suicidal plans. However, on the pertinent day, he could not carry on. He decided to commit suicide by slicing his wrists, but first he strangled his wife so that she would not stay behind alone and helplessly. The unannounced visit of his brother disturbed the plan, because he found the suspect unconscious and then called the alarm number. Intensive medical care saved the suspect's life, but his wife was dead.

Approximately 3 months later, in June, the suspect turned and testified that he had no clear recollection of what had happened. His defence elaborated this new content into a claim of amnesia. In this line of reasoning, the suspect had not killed his wife, but solely found her dead. She had died of cardiac arrest. Strikingly, post mortem medical examination did not deliver a clear cause of death, and left both a natural death and a murder scenario open. Upon finding his wife deceased, he tried to kill himself. When the police addressed him and woke him up, he must have confabulated that he killed his wife. In short, the evidence ended up much more ambiguously than anticipated initially. Several experts tried to shed light on this case.

ECLI:NL:RBZWB:2015:307

E. Rassin, *Case Studies in Legal Psychology*,
https://doi.org/10.1007/978-3-031-44931-4_10

10.1 Memory Enhancement

Although in the present case, no memory-enhancing techniques were applied, that would have been possible, particularly because the suspect was willing to cooperate. There are various techniques to improve the recollection of a specific event, all of which have a modest effect at best. One technique that was once proposed to improve recollection is hypnosis. During hypnosis, the witness (or in our case, the suspect) is brought in a state of attentional narrowing, in that he is focused on the voice of the interviewer. The goal is that this attentional narrowing increases concentration, and will hence improve retrieval performance. However, by now, it is assumed that forensic hypnosis has only limited positive effect on retrieval, while at the same time, it may well increase the number of falsely recalled details, especially if the interviewer were to (accidentally) pose leading questions (Kebbell & Wagstaff, 1998; Pinizzotto, 1989).

Another, simple, attempt to improve memory is to have the witness close his eyes in order to increase concentration. Perfect et al. (2008) showed participants a short film clip and asked them 15 questions about this film, with a do-not-know answer option. Some participants received a general free recall instruction, while others were additionally instructed to close their eyes during retrieval. Averaged over five studies, participants in the control condition answered 4.8 questions correctly, while those who closed their eyes were right 7 times. Interestingly, eye closure did not result in an increase of false answers with on average 2 in the control condition and 1.4 in the eyes closed condition.

Another technique to improve eyewitness recollection is the cognitive interview (CI; Geiselman et al., 1986). The CI includes, apart from optimal circumstances such as a quiet room, rapport building, and an uninterrupted interview, four approaches. First, the witness is instructed to mentally reinstate the context of the crime: Where was he standing, how was he feeling, and maybe even how was the weather? Second, the witness is instructed to report everything he remembers, even details he thinks are unimportant. These two instructions seek to retrieve as much information as possible. Note that details, even those that are not directly relevant may serve as retrieval cues for other details that are crucial to the police. Third, the witness may be asked to retell the event in an adapted chronology, for example backwardly. Fourth, the witness is instructed to retell the event from a different perspective, angle than his own. The latter two instructions specifically seek to suppress false details that may arise in a normal retrieval process in which mental scripts and expectations may be activated. A meta-analysis by Memon et al. (2010), covering 46 publications and 2887 participants, yielded a positive effect size ($d = 1.2$) for the recollection of correct details, but indeed also a (smaller) positive effect size ($d = 0.24$) for incorrect ones. The latter was excluding confabulations; these were analysed separately and were found to not increase significantly ($d = 0.08$; $p = 0.10$). Additional moderator analyses suggested that older adults benefit more from the CI than do young adults, but also that children, on average, benefit slightly less than young adults. Further, strong emotionality of the witnessed event suppressed the effect of the CI when compared with neutral events. Finally, with increases in delay between witnessed event and interview, the beneficiary effect of the CI on correct details decreases, whereas the relative number of confabulations increases. The latter suggests that, particularly from a legal psychological stance, the CI should not be used after a longer delay. Notably, the CI has been modified several times over the years. For example, additional instructions such as drawing a sketch of the crime scene and not guessing have been included.

A final example of a protocol directed at increasing eyewitness recall is the recently developed self-administered interview (SAI; Hope et al., 2011). Basic idea is that witnesses should be interviewed a soon as possible, to prevent loss of memory, to consolidate recollecting, and thus offer protection against later post event information, and to make police benefit most from witness information so as to optimize allocation of investigation means. The SAI is originally meant for situations in which a crime or accident (e.g., a terrorist attack, or a traffic accident) is witnessed by multiple witnesses. The idea is that the police hand out written SAI instructions to all witnesses present at the scene. SAI consists of seven separate instructions. (A) The free recall instruction includes several aspects that stem from the CI. The witness is first instructed to take time to reinstate the context in his mind ('Where were you, what were you doing, who were you with, how were you feeling, what was happening, who was involved, what could you see, and what could you hear?'). A report everything instruction is also included. (B) Second, the witness is instructed to describe the perpetrator in as much detail as possible. (C) The witness is asked to draw a sketch of the (crime) scene. (D) The witness is asked to describe any other witnesses he has seen. (E) Detailed descriptions of any vehicles present at or involved in the event are solicited. (F) Next, witnessing conditions are targeted, such as the weather, the time of day, lighting, distance, exposure duration, and possible obstructions. (G) Finally, the witness is asked to report any other information not covered by the previous instructions. The SAI is becoming increasingly popular, and while direct scientific scrutiny is scarce, on theoretical grounds, the SAI should be beneficial to eyewitness evidence.

10.2 Genuine or Simulated Amnesia

The prosecution did not take the claim of amnesia seriously. They believed it to be a strategy to dodge criminal responsibility. In this line of reasoning, the amnesia was simulated and the suspect lied about his memory loss. In theory, there are various approaches to detect deception, with different accuracy. In Chap. 5, verbal deception detection techniques such as CBCA were discussed. However, in case of claimed amnesia, such techniques offer little solution because there is not much content to analyse. An alternative approach would be to analyse the suspect's nonverbal behaviour when discussing his memory (loss). Unfortunately, though, the literature is not optimistic about the effect of relying on nonverbal cues on our detection accuracy. Wiseman (1995) interviewed a well-known political commentator, Sir Robin Day, on two occasions. On one occasion, Day truthfully talked about his favourite film, and on the other occasion, he pretended to talk about his favourite film, while actually talking about a film he disliked. Wiseman subjected the two fragments to 41,471 lay participants who judged which fragment was truthful and which was deceitful, without any special aids. Some participants were presented with the (audio-visual) film recording of the interview on tv. Others were presented with an audio version, by radio. The third group of participants were presented with a written version of the interviews, in a local newspaper. Interestingly, the newspaper readers achieved an accuracy rate of 64.2%, the radio listeners 73.4%, but the tv viewers no more than 51.8%. Apparently, adding audio cues increased the already impressive performance in case of written (verbal) presentation, but the visual cues were quite misleading. Hence, judges were better off with written than with audio-visual presentation. Bond and DePaulo (2006) conducted a meta-analysis on 206 articles, including 24,483 judges, and came up with an overall accuracy rate of 54% which is barely different from chance level. This disappointing accuracy level was made up of 61% accuracy at detecting truths, and 47% accuracy at detecting lies. Gongola et al. (2017) conducted a similar meta-analysis, but then specifically for the detection of lies in children. They included 45 experiments, covering 7892 adult judges and 1858 testifying children. These authors concluded that the average accuracy rate was 54%, with 63.8% truth detection accuracy, and 47.5% lie detection accuracy. Thus, we seem to be better at detecting truths than at detecting deceit. This may well be due to the fact that we have a preference to believe and are thus prone to gullibility. In other words, we may have a general truth bias.

In sum, there is good reason to argue that, when having access to audio-visual information, people are not accurate in their assessment of truthfulness. Research findings are also rather harsh on the idea that individuals differ in their capability to detect lies. Ekman and colleagues (1991, 1999) subjected various samples of participants to deception detection tests, using audio-visual presentations (i.e., film clips). Their performance is summarised in Table 10.1.

The findings appear to suggest that participants are poor at deception detection, yet slightly improved between 1991 and 1999. Further, the secret service samples appeared to perform relatively well. However, later meta-analyses rejected this idea. Aamodt and Custer (2006) included 108 studies, covering 16,537 participants, and

Table 10.1 Deception detection accuracy in various samples

	Ekman and O'Sullivan (1991)	Ekman et al. (1999)
Secret service	64.1%	73%
Polygraphers	55.7%	–
Police officers	55.8%	50.8%
Judges	56.7%	62%
Psychiatrists	57.6%	–
Students	52.8%	–
Sheriffs	–	66.7%
Clinical psychologists	–	62.1%

concluded that age, experience, education, gender, nor profession were associated with detection accuracy. Further, the authors argued that there is too little information to draw conclusions about the association with personality characteristics. Similarly, Bond and DePaulo (2008) reanalysed data from 247 samples and concluded that samples differ less than 1% in accuracy. They concluded: 'When judging deception, people differ less in ability than in the inclination to regard others' statements as truthful … Moreover, some people are more credible than others whether lying or truth telling … the outcome of a deception judgment depends more on the liar's credibility than any other individual difference' (p. 477).

The question arises how the poor performance can be explained. Vrij (2004) offers several theoretical accounts. First, there is no Pinocchio's nose. That is, no single cue corresponds perfectly with lying. This is so because there are various underlying processes that cause cues to occur. For example, there are various competing emotional processes that may be invoked by lying, such as nervousness or excitement. Obviously, nervousness will manifest in leaked cues that differ from those caused by positive excitement. Besides emotions, cognitive effort required to tell a convincing lie can result in the occurrence of specific cues. Note that these cognitive cues are mediated by factors such as preparation time, intelligence, and social expressiveness. Finally, attempts to control alleged cues (i.e., impression management) may paradoxically result in overcompensation producing cues to deception.

Second, the cues that do, imperfectly, correspond with deceit are rather small. Hence, they are difficult to detect, particularly, if, simultaneously, social rules of conversation are to be adhered to. Therefore, people miss the subtle cues to deception quite often. Hartwig and Bond (2011) argue that the subtlety of deception cues is a major cause of our poor performance at deception detection.

Third, not only are cues to deception rare and subtle, people tend to rely on subjective, false, nondiagnostic cues while ignoring the actual, objective cues to deception. DePaulo et al. (2003) conducted a meta-analysis on 158 potential cues to deception (verbal and nonverbal ones), and concluded that only 25 (i.e., 16%) were found to actually discriminate between true and false statements. These working cues were as follows.

1. Truths contain more information.
2. Truths contain more details.
3. Liars press their lips more.
4. Truths are more plausible.
5. Truths are more logically structured.
6. Liars behave more discrepant, ambivalent.
7. Liars display less verbal and vocal involvement.
8. Truth tellers display more illustrators (e.g., supporting hand movements).
9. Truth tellers are more verbally immediate.
10. Truth tellers are more verbally and vocally immediate (regarding impressions).
11. Liars express more verbal and vocal uncertainty.
12. Liars raise their chin more often.

13. Liars repeat themselves more often (on word and phrase level).
14. Truth tellers are more cooperative.
15. Liars make more negative statements and complaints.
16. Liars make more unpleasant faces.
17. Liars are more nervous and tensed.
18. Liars display more vocal tension.
19. Liars have a higher vocal pitch.
20. Liars' pupils are dilated.
21. Liars fidget more.
22. Truth tellers include more spontaneous corrections in their narratives.
23. Truth tellers more readily admit memory lacks.
24. Liars include more references to related external associations.
25. Liars display more response latency, but only if there was no preparation time.

Crucially, these cues are not only evident from experimental analogue studies, but also from field studies in which the narratives of actual witnesses and suspects were studied (see Vrij & Mann, 2001).

Fourth, besides the problems with the occurrence, magnitude, and detection of objective cues to detection, it must be acknowledged that lie detection is particularly difficult if the detector does not know the ground truth, which is often if not virtually always the case. Note that in most cases of deception detection, the observer is not only trying to find out whether the suspect is lying or speaking the truth, but simultaneously, what the truth is. Likewise, it remains to be seen how much effort the detector is really willing to invest in lie detection. In some instances, people may simply be satisfied with a superficial, standard scrutinization, in absence of a real, deep motivation to find fact. This is sometimes referred to as the ostrich effect (Vrij, 2004).

Fifth, and finally, judgements regarding deceit are hampered by the occurrence of various kinds of biases, especially if the judge has little knowledge to lean on. Vrij (2004) mentions the following. The expectancy violation heuristic predicts that observers will be overly tempted to judge behaviours that they seldomly see as suspect and thus as potential cues to deception. Similarly, deception judgements may be susceptible to the representative heuristic, that is, people may overgeneralise behaviours that they think to indicate deception (e.g., nervousness), and thus classify nervous yet truth-telling individuals as liars. Next, the probing heuristic dictates that people will be more confident in their veracity judgement after having had personal contact with the communicator. The facial appearance heuristic refers to the finding that attractive people and people with baby faces are generally believed more than average. People have also been found to believe their conversational partner more if they share the same accent (Lev-Ari & Keysar, 2010). In a study by Forgas and East (2008), participants were more trusting when in a good mood compared to when a sad mood had been induced by viewing a depressing film clip. Further, people tend to underestimate interindividual differences in behaviour, as well as intraindividual differences. The latter is referred to as the fundamental attribution error: In effect, we simply believe that some people are trustworthy and others are not, and thus, we ignore situational influences on deception.

Finally, as mentioned previously, our accuracy may be tempered by a fundamental truth bias. If we are indeed by nature prone to believe information, and given that some information is false, we are more likely to hold false (positive) beliefs than to not believe information that is in fact true. Hence, we are prone to suffer from gullibility (e.g., Forer, 1949; Meehl, 1956). Gilbert et al. (1990) offer an interesting account of truth bias. They tested two competing models of information processing. First, there is the Cartesian, intuitively plausible account. In this account, when being confronted with new information, we will first try to comprehend the information, and subsequently try to decide whether we believe it, or not. Hence, the Cartesian account includes two stages: (1) understanding and (2) acceptance or rejection. In the competing Spinozan account, the first stage of information processing comprises two inseparable processes, namely comprehension and acceptance. Thus, understanding and believing are virtually the same. What we understand, we by definition must believe, initially. In the second stage, we may decide to reject the information after all. While the Spinozan account may appear counterintuitive, its advantage is that processing new information is more efficient. That is, all new information that is understood is by default considered to be true. Only occasionally, a piece of information has to be rejected after all. This constellation of processes is more efficient than the Cartesian account in which one has to decide for each piece of information whether it is true or false. The efficiency inherent in the Spinozan account is traded off with an increase in false positive beliefs because, probably, not all falsity is detected in the second stage.

To test the Cartesian versus the Spinozan account, Gilbert et al. (1990) presented participants with new information, and rapidly interrupted the processing with a competing task. If the Cartesian account is correct, participants should be equally likely to believe or disbelieve the information. By contrast, if the Spinozan account is true, participants whose information processing is interrupted will end up believing more (partially processed) information than rejecting it. In their Hopi language experiment, Gilbert et al. sequentially presented 28 translations from Hopi to English (e.g., "a tarka is a wolf") to 35 female undergraduates. Immediately after each translation, participants were informed that the translation was actually correct or false. In some instances, this information processing of the veracity of the propositions was interrupted by a competing task in which participants had to press a specific button when they heard a noise. After this learning task, participants were given a memory task in which they had to recall whether or not a given translation was correct. On average, 55% of the correct translations were remembered as such by participants who had processed these without interruption. Similarly, 58% of the correct translations was remembered as such if the initial processing had been interrupted. However, uninterrupted incorrect translations were remembered as such in 55% of the cases, compared to 35% of the interrupted instances. Indeed, when interrupted, participants misremembered incorrect translations to be correct more often than vice versa. In another experiment, 71 female undergraduates read a crime story on screen (e.g., about Tom who robbed a stranger who gave him a ride, or about Kevin who robbed a convenience store; Gilbert et al., 1993). They were told that the story contained both correct information (printed in black) and false information

Table 10.2 Recognition performance in Gilbert et al. (1993)

	Uninterrupted		Interrupted
True statements recalled as true	93%		89%
True statements recalled as false	3%		6%
True statements recalled as foils	3%		4%
False statements recalled as true	23%	*	44%
False statements recalled as false	69%	*	34%
False statements recalled as foils	9%	*	23%
Foils recalled as true	5%	*	9%
Foils recalled as false	1%		5%
Foils recalled as foils	94%	*	86%

Note. * $p < 0.05$

(printed in red). Interruption took place when a blue-printed string of digits incidentally crawled by at the bottom of the screen. Whenever such a string appeared, participants had to press a button if there was a five present in the string. Eventually, participants underwent a recognition task in which they had to decide whether each of 30 statements were correct, false, or foils (not included in the story). Performances for the three kinds of statements, as a function of interruption, are presented in Table 10.2.

As can be seen, when interrupted, participants were less able to recognise false statements as such. This supports the Spinozan account of truth bias. However, there is also some critique on these studies by Gilbert and colleagues. For example, even without interruption, true statements were, at face value, more often identified as such (93%), than were false statements correctly identified (69%). If so, truth bias also occurs without interruption, and thus, the Spinozan account is not necessary for the occurrence of truth bias. Another critique is that the studies heavily rely on memory, but are silent about initial impressions of truth and falsity (Nadarevic & Erdfelder, 2013). In addition, the paradigms do not allow participants to opt for a do-not-know option. Such an option may make the truth bias disappear (Street & Kingstone, 2016; Street & Richardson, 2015).

The disappointing findings concerning our capacity to judge veracity has invited researchers to find ways to improve deception detection performance. One obvious strategy would be training. Driskell (2012) conducted a meta-analysis on 16 studies of deception detection training and found a small but significant positive effect ($d = 0.5$). Crucially, for a training to be effective, it needs to include transfer of correct theoretical knowledge, practice opportunity, and feedback. An example of a deception detection training programme that may fall short on the criterion that sound theory should be taught to trainees is the one included in the book of Inbau et al. (2001). This American police training book is notorious under researchers, because it is almost solely directed at gathering evidence against the suspect, and virtually ignores to possibility that the suspect might be innocent after all. In this book, several cues to deception are promoted that are not on the list produced by DePaulo et al. (2003) and are probably not diagnostic, such as gaze aversion and

Table 10.3 Findings by Kassin and Fong (1999), and Meissner and Kassin (2002)

	Naive		Trained	Police officers
Test score (0–20)	5.8	*	13.3	–
Accuracy (0–8)	4.4 (56%)	*	3.7 (46%)	4.0 (50%)
Confidence (1–10)	5.9	*	6.6	7.1

Note. * $p < 0.05$

posture changing. Kassin and Fong (1999) had students commit a mock crime, or not, and had them subsequently interrogated by police detective McCarthy. All students (whether guilty of the mock crime or not) were instructed that they would receive extra financial reward if they successfully convinced McCarthy that they were innocent. At some point during the 5 min interrogation, detective McCarthy said: 'Dammit, you were caught red-handed, so stop lying to me. I want to know exactly, minute by minute, where you were and what you were doing before you were picked up' (Kassin & Fong, 1999, p. 504). The interrogations were videotaped, and eight of them were later shown to participants. Twenty participants underwent a training based on the Inbau et al. (2001) book prior to viewing the fragments, while 20 others took up the veracity judgements naively. All participants made a 20 items test about the book (as a manipulation check), rated the eight interrogation fragments on the veracity of the suspects' denials, and rated the confidence in their own performance. Findings are displayed in Table 10.3. As can be seen, undergoing the Inbau et al. (2001), training made observers actually worse at deception detection, even though they felt more confident about their performance. Meissner and Kassin (2002) conducted the same experiment in a sample of police officers and obtained virtually the same findings (see Table 10.3, final column).

A simple way to employ the correct objective cues to deception is what Vrij (2004) called implicit or indirect lie detection. In this approach, one should not wonder whether one's conversation partner is lying, but whether, for example, he is making few illustrators. This alternative, indirect focus prevents the observer from relying on nondiagnostic cues.

Besides training in deception detection, training in interview techniques might also be fruitful in raising deception detection accuracy. For one thing, it seems important to learn to refrain from confronting one's partner with inconsistencies, because such a confrontation is likely to stop him talking and to become alerted that his credibility is under fire. It is better to have him talk more because this increases the probability that he will get entangled in the web of lies (Vrij, 2004). It has also been proposed to use cognitive interventions (cf. cognitive lie detection, e.g., by imposing cognitive load, encouraging the interviewee to report everything, eliciting the testimony in a changed order or perspective, and asking unexpected questions) as a magnifying glass, enlarging the differences between truthful and deceitful narratives (Vrij, 2018). Based on a meta-analysis of 14 studies, Vrij et al. (2017) argue that cognitive lie detection can increase deception detection accuracy from 56% in the control conditions to 71% in the CI conditions.

Another way to improve deception detection accuracy is to combine various types of cues. Whereas scientific research neatly distinguishes verbal from nonverbal deception detection, in real life, there may be much more information available to judges, including both kinds of cues, and multiple cues anyway. The combination of multiple cues is considered to increase accuracy (Vrij & Mann, 2004). Based on a meta-analysis comprising 26,866 narratives communicated by 9380 senders, Hartwig and Bond (2014) even argue that the combination of cues can increase accuracy to nearly 70%, which is impressive given the literature on deception detection accuracy.

One final, theoretically crucial improvement is that deception detection methods should include baselines. This means that the scores of particular narratives or observed communicators on any detection measure should be compared to a baseline, before any conclusion about veracity is drawn. Unfortunately, absolute baselining is virtually impossible, because clear cut-off scores are lacking for any criterion (Vrij, 2016). However, instead of using absolute baselines, judges could rely on relative baselines. For example, when using CBCA, observes could not only score the to-be-evaluated narrative but also score a comparable narrative by the same witness (e.g., a narrative about an emotional unrelated event, such as an unpleasant dental treatment) and compare both scores. In this way, scores become more meaningful. In fact, it is rather dubious that such baselines are not standardly included in deception detection instruments. Indeed, in their meta-analysis, Bond and DePaulo (2006) found that prior familiarity with the sender, increases the receiver's accuracy from 52% to 56%.

While the police, prosecution, and judges may well have formed an impression about the suspect's credibility based on his nonverbal behaviour, the current case would have allowed for a very specific, and fairly diagnostic technique. The basic idea behind this so-called symptom validity testing (SVT) is that the behaviour of the test subject is scrutinized by comparison of what might be expected of him. This approach stems from neuropsychology (Pankratz, 1979). Imagine that a patient claims to suffer from amnesia, but the treating psychologists suspects that the patient may simulate or exaggerate his complaints, for example because the patient may have an ulterior motive to feign amnesia. In such a situation, the psychologist may do a provocation test to measure the sincerity of the complaints. An example is Rey's 15 items test (see Lezak, 1983). In this test, the patient is told that he will undergo a difficult memory test to measure the severity of his amnesia. He is then presented with the card displayed in Fig. 10.1, for a few seconds, and instructed to try to memorise all the items on the card, ostensibly a difficult task.

The card is then taken away, and the patient is instructed to recall all items. People with genuine amnesia will still be able to recall at least eight items. However, some simulating amnestics may overdo their complaints and recall less than eight digits. Such an improbably poor performance indicates that the patient is likely simulating or exaggerating his complaints. Hence, this kind of provocation test seeks to lure the test subject into betraying himself by displaying improbable behaviour. Crucially, this approach is only possible if the ground truth (e.g., how do genuine memory problems manifest) is known. Besides symptom validity performance

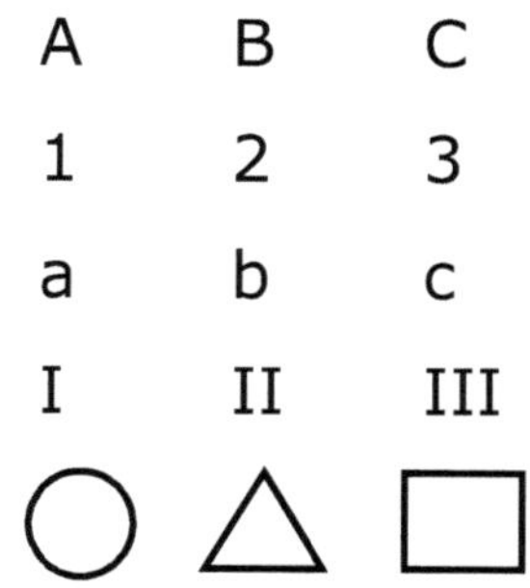

Fig. 10.1 Rey's 15 items test

test, the principle can also be applied to self-reports, by testing whether the subject endorses complaints that are generally not typical of the syndrome that he claims to suffer from (e.g., Crowne & Marlow, 1960; Rubenzer, 2022; Smith & Burger, 1997). Oftentimes, symptom validity tests are neatly specific, but less sensitive, because test subjects see through the test and manage to fake symptoms well. As to Rey's 15 items test, Boone et al. (2002) managed to increase sensitivity to 71% while maintaining a specificity of 92%, by adding a recognition test.

Denney (1996) sought to apply this principle to autobiographical recollections. Imagine that a suspect (or witness) claims to never have been at the crime scene. If this suspect were to be subjected to a memory test about the crime scene consisting of 20 forced choice yes/no questions (e.g., 'Was the crime committed indoors?'), it is to be expected that he would accidentally answer approximately 10 items correct. That is, $N = 20$, and $p = 0.5$ (and 20 * 0.5 = 10). Now, imagine that the suspect actually was at the crime scene, and therefore only pretends not knowing the answers to the 20 questions. Imagine further that he overdoes his acted ignorance and answers significantly less than 10 items correctly. If so, the psychologist can conclude that the suspect actually knows the answers and purposely underperforms. Denney (1996) presented a simple formula to compute whether a specific performance is at chance level or below. This formula is as follows:

$$-z = x - N\,p\,/\,\sqrt{\left(N\,p\left(1-p\right)\right)}.$$

In this formula, N stands for the total number of questions, p for the probability of answering a question correctly by chance, and x for the number of questions answered correctly. The computed Z-score can be used to find the corresponding p-value. Generally, a Z-score of (−)1.65 is significant at $p = 0.05$, and a Z-score of (−)2.33 is significant at $p = 0.01$. In the current example, four or less correctly answered items would be so improbably that it can be concluded that the suspect is feigning. Reiterate that in this approach, the ground truth is in fact known to the psychologist. The goal of the test is merely to find out whether the witness/suspect is lying.

Merckelbach et al. (2002) had 20 undergraduates commit a mock crime (i.e., to steel an envelope from a lab room), and subjected them to a 15-item SVT, under the instruction that they were to feign amnesia for their visit to the room. Six participants (i.e., 30%) performed at chance level (i.e., between 5 and 10 correct answers), six performed above chance level (i.e., >11 correct answers), and eight (i.e., 40%) performed below chance level (i.e., <4 correct answers). These findings are silent about the selectivity of this SVT procedure, but suggest that its sensitivity is modest. Note that 70% of simulating participants were exposed: 40% because they were provoked to perform below chance level, and 30% because they directly failed to perform below their knowledge.

10.3 A Small Battle of Forensic Experts

In this case, quite a few experts were consulted. It is also interesting to see that the matter of amnesia is at a cross point between legal and forensic psychology. Even under the prosecution's primary hypothesis, there was reason to call upon psychological (and psychiatric) expertise. Not because of a distrust of the suspect's confession, but because of a suspected reduction in criminal responsibility. To assess the suspects mental health, he was evaluated by a forensic psychologist, Dr. Vuister, and a forensic psychiatrist, Dr. Trompenaars. The former subjected the suspect to various tests, including an intelligence test, the MMPI, a psychodynamic sentence completion test, and a risk assessment instrument (HCR-20). By and large, this expert came to the conclusion that the suspect had an average-low intelligence, a low risk of recidivism, and no apparent psychiatric disturbances. The psychiatrist did not subject the suspect to any tests, but had two meetings with him. He confirmed the diagnoses of the psychologist, and both concluded that the suspect's criminal responsibility was in no way suppressed. Neither of these two experts mentioned any signs of memory problems. Admittedly though, their assignment was to diagnose the suspect's criminal responsibility for the murder, whereas the alleged memory problems only arose after the killing (or better: after finding the dead body of his wife).

Under the alternative hypothesis of the defence, two concerns were crucial, namely the memory loss and the confabulated confession. Further, the absence of clear traces of strangulation played an important role in the line of defence. A forensic medical examiner, Dr. Kubat, reported that the woman had suffered from various life-threatening abnormalities of her heart. The expert also reported that the absence of strangulation marks (cf. negative evidence) cannot be taken as evidence against strangulation. Nonetheless, the defence lawyer forwarded the hypothesis that the suspect had found his wife dead, got overwhelmed, and tried to kill himself. When he was rescued and saw his dead wife, he confabulated that he had killed her, but months later this confabulated confession did not seem to be accompanied by lasting recollections, and hence, he started reporting amnesia for the crime. The defence asked a legal psychologist, Dr. van Oorsouw, for her opinion on the validity of the confession and of the subsequent amnesia claim. This expert subjected the suspect to various tests in order to test the alternative hypothesis. The battery included eight DRM-lists. In all eight instances, the suspect falsely recognized the critical lure, which made the expert conclude that he had increased susceptibility to confabulation. The initial amnesia could be organic, that is, caused by massive blood loss, according to the expert. The expert also subjected the suspect to a symptom validity test, the Structured Inventory of Malingered Symptomatology (SIMS; Smith & Burger, 1997), on which he scored high enough to not be suspected of feigning his amnesia. In short, van Oorsouw concluded that there was some evidence for the alternative hypothesis in which amnesia due to blood loss and a false confession due to confabulation played a role.

The opinions of the respective experts differed vastly. Therefore, the court asked Vuister and Trompenaars explicitly whether they had seen signs of memory problems. Both experts stuck to their initial findings which did not include memory problems. The court appointed a second medical examiner to comment on van Oorsouw's claim about organic memory loss. This expert, Dr. Botter, saw no scientific argument for that claim. Particularly, he testified that our body has mechanisms to ensure that the most crucial organs (such as heart and brain) will keep functioning in case of damages. Therefore, organic memory loss should not occur if the individual is still half-conscious (as the suspect was).

The court also asked me two questions, namely whether in my opinion, the suspect's confession was false, and whether van Oorsouw's exposé on amnesia was accurate. As to the former topic, I referred to a study by Kassin and Kiechel (1996). They were the first to develop an experimental design with the pretence of modelling an interrogation. They had 79 undergraduates participate in a reaction time experiment. In this set-up, a second participant (in fact, a confederate) read aloud a list of letters, while the participant had to type these in on a computer key board as fast as possible. Participants were explicitly instructed not to press the alt key, because that would cause the software to crash, and the data to get lost. Approximately 1 min after the experiment had begun, the computer crashed. Upon this ordeal, the experimenter would ask the participant whether he had pressed the alt key. In fact, the software would always crash after 1 min, and none of the participants had actually pressed the alt key. Hence, admitting to have pressed the alt key would constitute a false confession. The experimenter asked participants to sign a written statement 'I hit the alt key and caused the program to crash. Data were lost'. The consequence would be that the participant was to expect a phone call from the principal investigator.

The crucial variable was how many participants would sign the written confession, thereby admitting to have done something that was forbidden and that would have potentially adverse consequences. Two extra variables were included. First, some participants were randomly allocated to the slow condition, in which the confederate read aloud approximately 43 letters per minute. Others were in the fast condition, in which the confederate read aloud 67 letters per minute. Second, when the experimenter asked whether the confederate had seen anything, she would sometimes reply that she had seen nothing. In other instances, she would reply that she had seen that the participant had indeed pressed the alt key. This latter response constitutes (false) incriminating eyewitness evidence.

Table 10.4 Confession rates in Kassin and Kiechel (1996)

	No witness statement		Incriminating witness statement		
	Slow	Fast	Slow	Fast	Overall
Signed confession	35%	65%	89%	100%	69%
Internalisation	0%	12%	44%	65%	28%
Confabulation	0%	0%	6%	35%	9%

After the participants left the lab, there was another person waiting outside. This person overheard the participant and the experimenter talk, and asked the participant what had happened. In reality, this person was also a stooge. The conversation between this stooge and the participant was recorded, and was used to find out why the participant had signed the confession (if he had done so). Finally, the experimenter returned, took the participant back to the lab, read aloud all letters typed in by the participant, and asked if they could reconstruct why they had pressed the alt key. From this final discussion, possible confabulations could be derived, that is, would participants make up reasons for having pressed the alt key, while they had not? Findings are summarised in Table 10.4. As can be seen, false confession rates were strikingly high, and contingent upon pace and confrontation with (false) evidence.

As an initial experimental study of the likelihood of eliciting false confessions, the alt key study (Kassin & Kiechel, 1996) has become a classic. By now, it has been replicated in various adapted designs. Rassin and Israëls (2014) conducted a review of 16 experiments in the vein of the alt key study. In all, there were 340 guilty participants in the experiments, of which 252 confessed (i.e., 74%). Of the 1559 innocent participants, no less than 707 falsely confessed (i.e., 45%). Consequently, the overall likelihood ratio of confession evidence would be (74%: 45% = 1.64) less than 2.

Based on this research, I concluded that the overall true positive likelihood of a confession is around 74%, while the likelihood of a false confession with confabulated details is about 9%, that is, after suggestive questioning, which was absent in the present case. Hence, I estimated the likelihood of the confession being true to be 8 to 10 times higher than that the confession was false. In hindsight, I framed my conclusion inappropriately, because it suffered from a prosecutor's fallacy. I should not have addressed the likelihood of the confession being true or false, but merely the likelihood of giving a true or false confession.

As to the court's second question, I replied that I had insufficient pertinent knowledge to give an opinion on the organic amnesia due to blood loss. I also did not know whether blood loss will result in anterograde amnesia (i.e., being unable to remember new happenings) or retrograde amnesia (i.e., being unable to remember events before the blood loss). Finally, I stressed that in my opinion, the absence of amnesia in the reports of the forensic psychologist and psychiatrist did not support the primary hypothesis, because these experts did not, and did not have to look for amnesia.

Eventually, the court was not convinced of the alternative account of organic amnesia and the confabulated false confession. The suspect was convicted to 10 years of imprisonment. That verdict was confirmed in appeal.

References

Aamodt, M. G., & Custer, H. (2006). Who can best catch a liar? A meta-analysis of individual differences in detecting deception. *The Forensic Examiner, Spring Issue*, 6–11.

Bond, C. F., & DePaulo, B. M. (2006). Accuracy of deception judgments. *Personality and Social Psychology Review, 10*, 214–234.

Bond, C. F., & DePaulo, B. M. (2008). Individual differences in judging deception: Accuracy and bias. *Psychological Bulletin, 134*, 477–492.

Boone, K. B., Salazar, X., Lu, P., Warner-Chacon, K., & Razani, J. (2002). The Rey 15-item recognition trial: A technique to enhance sensitivity of the Rey 15-item memorization test. *Journal of Clinical and Experimental Neuropsychology, 24*(5), 561–573.

Crowne, D. P., & Marlowe, D. (1960). A new scale of social desirability independent of psychopathology. *Journal of Consulting Psychology, 24*, 349–354.

Denney, R. L. (1996). Symptom validity testing of remote memory in a criminal forensic setting. *Archives of Clinical Neuropsychology, 11*, 589–603.

DePaulo, B. M., Lindsay, J. J., Malone, B. E., Muhlenbruck, L., Charlton, K., & Cooper, H. (2003). Cues to deception. *Psychological Bulletin, 129*, 74–118.

Driskell, J. E. (2012). Effectiveness of deception detection training: A meta-analysis. *Psychology, Crime & Law, 18*, 713–731.

Ekman, P., & O'Sullivan, M. (1991). Who can catch a liar? *American Psychologist, 46*, 913–920.

Ekman, P., O'Sullivan, M., & Frank, M. G. (1999). A few can catch a liar. *Psychological Science, 10*, 263–266.

Forer, B. R. (1949). The fallacy of personal validation: A classroom demonstration of gullibility. *Journal of Abnormal and Social Psychology, 44*, 118–123.

Forgas, J. P., & East, R. (2008). On being happy and gullible: Mood effects on skepticism and the detection of deception. *Journal of Experimental Social Psychology, 44*, 1362–1367.

Geiselman, R. E., Fisher, R. P., MacKinnon, D. P., & Holland, H. L. (1986). Enhancement of eyewitness memory with the cognitive interview. *American Journal of Psychology, 99*, 385–401.

Gilbert, D. T., Krull, D. S., & Malone, P. S. (1990). Unbelieving the unbelievable: Some problems in the rejection of false information. *Journal of Personality and Social Psychology, 59*, 601–613.

Gilbert, D. T., Tafarodi, R. W., & Malone, P. S. (1993). You can't not believe anything you read. *Journal of Personality and Social Psychology, 65*, 221–233.

Gongola, J., Scurich, N., & Quas, J. A. (2017). Detecting deception in children: A meta-analysis. *Law and Human Behavior, 41*, 44–54.

Hartwig, M., & Bond, C. F. (2011). Why do lie-catchers fail? A lens model meta-analysis of human lie judgments. *Psychological Bulletin, 137*, 643–659.

Hartwig, M., & Bond, C. F. (2014). Lie detection from multiple cues: A meta-analysis. *Applied Cognitive Psychology, 28*, 661–676.

Hope, L., Gabbert, F., & Fisher, R. P. (2011). From laboratory to the street: Capturing witness memory using the self-administered interview. *Legal and Criminological Psychology, 16*, 211–226.

Inbau, F. E., Reid, J. E., Buckley, J. P., & Jayne, B. C. (2001). *Criminal interrogation and confessions*. Aspen Publishers.

Kassin, S. M., & Fong, C. T. (1999). "I'm innocent!" Effects of training on judgments of truth and deception in the interrogation room. *Law and Human Behavior, 23*, 499–516.

Kassin, S. M., & Kiechel, K. L. (1996). The social psychology of false confessions: Compliance, internalization, and confabulation. *Psychological Science, 7*, 125–128.
Kebbell, M. R., & Wagstaff, G. F. (1998). Hypnotic interviewing: The best way to interview eyewitnesses? *Behavioral Sciences & the Law, 16*, 115–129.
Lev-Ari, S., & Keysar, B. (2010). Why don't we believe non-native speakers? The influence of accent on credibility. *Journal of Experimental Social Psychology, 46*, 1093–1096.
Lezak, M. D. (1983). *Neuropsychological assessment*. Oxford university press.
Meehl, P. E. (1956). Wanted – A good cookbook. *American Psychologist, 11*, 263–272.
Meissner, C. A., & Kassin, S. M. (2002). "He's guilty!": Investigator bias in judgments of truth and deception. *Law and Human Behavior, 26*, 469–480.
Memon, A., Meissner, C. A., & Fraser, J. (2010). The cognitive interview: A meta-analytic review and study space analysis of the past 25 years. *Psychology, Public Policy, and Law, 16*, 340–372.
Merckelbach, H., Hauer, B., & Rassin, E. (2002). Symptom validity testing of feigned dissociative amnesia: A simulation study. *Psychology, Crime & Law, 8*, 311–318.
Nadarevic, L., & Erdfelder, E. (2013). Spinoza's error: Memory for truth hand falsity. *Memory and Cognition, 41*, 176–186.
Pankratz, L. (1979). Symptom validity testing and symptom retraining: Procedures for the assessment and treatment of functional sensory deficits. *Journal of Consulting and Clinical Psychology, 47*, 409–410.
Perfect, T. J., Wagstaff, G. F., Moore, D., Andrews, B., Cleveland, V., Newcombe, S., Brisbane, K. A., & Brown, L. (2008). How can we help witnesses to remember more? It's an (eyes) open and shut case. *Law and Human Behavior, 32*, 314–324.
Pinizzotto, A. J. (1989). Memory and hypnosis: Implications for the use of forensic hypnosis. *Professional Psychology: Research and Practice, 20*, 322–328.
Rassin, E., & Israëls, H. (2014). False confessions in the lab: A review. *Erasmus Law Review, 7*, 219–224.
Rubenzer, S. J. (2022). Ruling out feigned crime-related amnesia? A response to Acklin, *Behavioral Science and the Law*, 1–17. https://doi.org/10.1002/bsl.2623
Smith, G. P., & Burger, G. K. (1997). Detection of malingering: Validation of the structured inventory of malingered symptomatology (SIMS). *Journal of the Academy of Psychiatry and the Law, 25*, 183–190.
Street, C. N. H., & Kingstone, A. (2016). Aligning Spinoza with Descartes: An informed Cartesian account of the truth bias. *British Journal of Psychology, 108*, 453–466.
Street, C. N. H., & Richardson, D. C. (2015). Descartes versus Spinoza: Truth, uncertainty, and bias. *Social Cognition, 33*, 227–239.
Vrij, A. (2004). Why professionals fail to catch liars and how they can improve. *Legal and Criminological Psychology, 9*, 159–181.
Vrij, A. (2016). Baselining as a lie detection method. *Applied Cognitive Psychology, 30*, 1112–1119.
Vrij, A. (2018). Deception and truth detection when analyzing nonverbal and verbal cues. *Applied Cognitive Psychology, 33*, 160–167.
Vrij, A., & Mann, S. (2001). Telling and detecting lies in a high-stake situation: The case of a convicted murderer. *Applied Cognitive Psychology, 15*, 187–203.
Vrij, A., & Mann, S. (2004). Detecting deception: The benefit of looking at a combination of behavioral, auditory and speech content cues in a systematic manner. *Group Decision and Negotiation, 13*, 61–79.
Vrij, A., Fisher, R. P., & Blank, H. (2017). A cognitive approach to lie detection: A meta-analysis. *Legal and Criminological Psychology, 22*, 1–21.
Wiseman, R. (1995). The megalab truth test. *Nature, 373*, 391.

Chapter 11
The Breda Six

In the morning of Sunday July 4, 1993 at 11:00 h, 56-year-old 'grandma' Mok is found dead in her Chinese restaurant Peacock in Breda. Medical examination shows that she was strangled between midnight and 6:00 h. From the crime scene, money and jewels are stolen, and a gambling machine is broken. It seems that miss Mok was killed by someone who burgled the restaurant on the night of 3–4 July. The police investigation remains fruitless and is closed on September 9 1993. But on March 18, 1994, the police receive a tip about six people, all in their early twenties: Appie, Ahmed, Anil, Jane, Jenny, and Carien. All suspects are interrogated repeatedly and intensely. The three men deny, but the three women eventually confess that they kidnapped miss Mok from her home and brought her to the restaurant by car in order to steal valuables. In their confessions, the women incriminate the three male suspects. The crime was allegedly committed by the six suspects conjointly. In fact, the men had come up with the idea in the first place. And it were the men who eventually killed the victim, because they wanted to prevent that she would describe them to the police and thus contribute to their arrest.

In 1994 and 1995, the six suspects are convicted for this crime. The men are sentenced to approximately 10 years of imprisonment. The women to less than 2 years. Meanwhile, the case has caught media attention. Also, the women have by now retracted their confessions, and claim that they had merely confessed because of police coercion and trickery. Legal psychologist Dr. van Koppen requested a special committee installed by the Supreme court to reopen the case. On behalf of this committee, advocate-general Aben presented nine nova (i.e., new insights that justify reopening of the case). One of these pertained to the retraction of the confessions. The Supreme Court gave its verdict in 2017. All suspects had served their imprisonment by then.

ECLI:NL:HR:2017:3189

E. Rassin, *Case Studies in Legal Psychology*,
https://doi.org/10.1007/978-3-031-44931-4_11

11.1 Interrogation

It is important to realise that the police are convinced that the suspect is involved in the crime when they decide to employ an interrogation protocol. This conviction and the protocol itself result in some pressure being inevitable. This is more so if the suspect denies. In the words of Inbau et al. (2001): 'Indeed, it is a rare occurrence when a guilty person, after being presented with a direct confrontation of guilt says: "Okay, you've got me; I did it." Almost always, the suspect, whether innocent or guilty, will initially make a denial' (p. 303). Possibly the best known trick to make silent, unwilling suspects talk, is the good cop bad cop approach, also known as Mutt and Jeff (Gudjonsson, 2003). In this approach, a couple of interrogators play distinct roles: One is the unsympathetic, and the other the relatively friendly one. At some point during the interrogation, the unsympathetic interrogator leaves the interrogation room. At this point, the sympathetic interrogator tries to get into contact with the suspect. The idea is that the suspect is more likely to talk then because the unsympathetic police officer has left the room.

Inbau et al. (2001) described a more elaborated protocol to make suspects talk, called the Reid nine steps of interrogation. The nine steps do not always have to be taken, and not necessarily in subsequent order anyway. When discussing this method, it has to be kept in mind, that it will be used once the police is convinced that the suspect is guilty. The first step is the direct positive confrontation. This means that it has to be made clear to the suspect that the police is indeed positively convinced that the suspect is guilty of the pertinent crime. It also has to be made clear that the police will continue interrogating the suspect until he confesses. With this positive confrontation, the police may intimidate the suspect, and convince him to confess right away. After the confrontation, a short behavioural pause should be taken, during which the interrogator places his file on the table, and awaits the reaction of the suspect. Generally, innocent suspects, if any, will react in a direct, aggressive way and deny any involvement straightforwardly: 'You're wrong, You've got to be crazy if you think I did something like that!' (Inbau et al., 2001, p. 314). By contrast, a guilty suspect will try to stall for time by asking rhetorical questions or make bolstered denials: 'Why do you think I did that?', 'Honestly sir, I've been telling you the truth', 'On my mother's grave', 'I knew this would happen', 'You're just out to get me. I'm framed' (p. 315).

The second step is theme development. The purpose of this step is to find an approach to communicate with the suspect in a way that opens the suspect to discussing the crime. Which approach works depends on whether the suspect is emotional or nonemotional. Themes that may well work with emotional suspects are third-person themes. For example, the interrogator may show sympathy for the suspect and say that anyone else under similar conditions would have done the same. Another theme is the minimisation of the moral seriousness of the offence. A third approach is to offer a morally more acceptable motive for the crime, than the one presumed. Fourth, the interrogator may try to condemn other parties involved, such as the victim or bystanders. By shifting blame to third parties, the suspect may be more willing to admit his involvement. A fifth theme is to appeal to the suspect's pride and urge him to accept the consequences of his actions. Sixth, the interrogator may try to make the impression that the victim's allegation is exaggerated. The seventh theme is to convince the suspect that continuation of his criminal behaviour and attitude (including his denial) is futile and will have serious consequences. If none of these themes work, the suspect may be nonemotional, and the interrogator should explore the harsher tactics, such as inflating the diagnosticity of a small lie or inconsistency in the suspect's testimony. Likewise, it is important to mentally place the suspect at the crime scene and in contact with the victim. Another approach is to suggest a noncriminal intent for the offence. Also, stressing the futility of denying, by claiming that there is already enough evidence to convict the suspect, may persuade the suspect to confess. If there are more suspects, they can be played one against the other, for example, by claiming that the other suspect already confessed and testified that his role was minor compared to that of the suspect. In effect, with this tactic, the interrogator lies to the suspect.

Step three concerns the handling of denials. According to Inbau et al. (2001), virtually all suspects will initially deny, after the direct positive confrontation. Weak denials should be ignored, so as to imply that the interrogator 'will not even waste his breath by responding to it' (p. 306). If a forceful denial is uttered, the interrogator should reiterate that there is a lot of evidence that clearly implicates the suspect. The guilty suspect will now understand that denying is futile. The innocent suspect, if any, will be more motivated to prove the interrogator wrong. The book does not say how he can do that. If the interrogator foresees denials later on, during theme development, he may prevent them from being uttered with nonverbal behaviour, such as raising his hand and making a stop sign. In addition, he should reiterate that it is completely clear that the suspect is guilty, and should then return to the theme at hand.

Step four is to overcome objections. Once a guilty suspect is beginning to understand that denials are futile, he may change his strategy to formulating objections (e.g., 'It is impossible that I would do something like that', 'I do not even own a gun'). It is important that the interrogator does not reject the objection right away, and will thus be drawn into a yes-no-argument. Instead, he should acknowledge the objection and turn it around (e.g., 'Of course you would not do something like that, and the fact that you do not have a gun tells me that you did not plan this. Perhaps it was someone else's idea … someone who does own a gun'). With this approach, it is possible to return to the theme swiftly.

Step five is the retention of the suspect's attention. At some point, the suspect will begin to understand that there is no other way out than confessing his crime. This realisation will cause the suspect to think hard, and to withdraw from the interrogation. It is then crucial to maintain the suspect's attention and to keep him involved. Literally moving closer to the suspect (chair proximity) is one technique to maintain attention. It is also important to establish eye contact. Further, the interrogator may bring physical evidence to the table (e.g., the weapon used in the crime, or a footprint; this may even be fake evidence).

Step six is called the handling of the suspect's passive mood, and is actually nothing more than an analysis of the suspect's (nonverbal) behaviour. The suspect is likely to resign, and this may show in a change in posture (e.g., keeping his head down and staring at the flour, nonverbally agreeing with the summary provided by the interrogator). It is important that the interrogator speaks slowly and empathically at this point.

Step seven is presenting an alternative question. In this step, the interrogator should provide an alternative motive for the crime, a motive that is more morally acceptable than the motive suspected by the police. This alternative motive should be the final incentive for the suspect to confess. The alternative question (1) should not refer to legal consequences of confessing (leniencies) or denying (threats), (2) should imply that the suspect is indeed guilty, (3) should build on the theme to which the suspect seemed most responsive, (4) should be presented in a leading manner (e.g., 'It was for your family's sake, wasn't it Joe?'; Inbau et al., 2001, p. 360), and (5) should reward the offered alternative motive and should express a negative evaluation of possible other motives (e.g., 'If that's why you did this, I don't even want to talk further because it means I've really misread you today!', p. 359).

In the eighth step, the interrogator should elicit as many crime-related details as possible from the suspect, in order to make the confession more elaborate and convincing. This can be achieved by rewarding each detail given by the suspect 'Good, that's what I thought it was all along … I was hoping that was the case', Inbau et al., 2001, p. 366). It is advisable that a second police officer is brought into the interrogation room, because the perceived presence of this witness reduces the suspect's tendency to withdraw the confession later on.

Step nine: The oral confession should be transcribed into a solid written and signed confession as soon as possible. It is important that the written confession includes that the suspect was informed about his constitutional rights. It should contain personal, specific details in order to appear tailor-made. Further 'it is a good practice to purposefully arrange for the inclusion, on each page of the confession, one or two errors, such as an incorrect name of a person or street, which will be subject to later correction by the confessor when the document is read by or to him. Any such correction should be in the confessor's own handwriting, accompanied by his initials or signature in the margin alongside the corrections. When confronted at the trial with a confession bearing corrections of this nature, the confessor will encounter considerable difficulty in denying having read the document before signing it' (Inbau et al., 2001, p. 383–384).

In sum, the Reid nine steps of interrogation is a protocol aimed at making guilty suspects confess (Inbau et al., 2001). Kassin (1997) summarises the approach as a combination of maximising disadvantages and anxiety associated with denying (= lying), while minimising perceived negative consequences of confessing by inducing a false sense of security. Many academic authors are quite critical about this protocol, because it is one-sidedly focused on obtaining a confession, rather than on fact finding. Consequently, the interrogation technique is feared to result in false confessions (e.g., Gudjonsson, 2003; Kassin, 1997, 2005). In addition, the technique includes some tricks that are arguably dubious. For example, as mentioned, the interrogator may present false evidence to the suspect. Hence, this constitutes lying. Moreover, according to some authors, it may push innocent suspects towards making a false confession. This fear is not commonly shared by the police. In response to expressing this possibility, Kassin (2005) usually receives the following reaction: 'No, because I do not interrogate innocent people' (p. 216). Inbau et al. (2001) argue in general terms: 'None of what is recommended is apt to induce an innocent person to offer a confession' (p. 313), and: 'It is our contention, however, that an innocent suspect operating within normal limits of competency would not accept physical responsibility for an act he knows he did not commit' (p. 286). With respect to the advice to occasionally lie to the suspect, they argue: 'The important question to answer is whether it is human nature to accept responsibility for something we did not do in the face of contrary evidence. Upon checking a sales receipt a customer may discover that the clerk rang up the same item twice. Under this circumstance, certainly the customer would challenge the evidence (the sales receipt) rather than pay for something not purchased … The ordinary citizen is outraged and indignant when presented with supposed "evidence" of an act he knows he did not commit' (p. 428).

Within the Reid nine steps of interrogation protocol, it is also allowed to make false promises and threats. For example, it is always considered permissible to tell the suspect that he will feel better after confessing, that his peers will have respect for him confessing his crime and that he will personally grow and prevent himself from making similar mistakes in the future, by confessing. These promises are lies in the sense that the interrogator has no way of knowing what the psychological consequences of confessing will be. Indeed, there is little reason to argue that a confession will bring any relief to the suspect. Inbau et al. (2001) caution the interrogator that threats and promises regarding legal consequences of confessing and denying should be used sensibly. The reason to be prudent with these is not that they are somehow unethical, but merely that their use can be counterproductive, in that a well-informed suspect may call the bluff, and/or the judge may consider the confession to be weaker if these kinds of promises and threats have preceded. Interestingly, research suggests that while participants perceive confessions that result from promises equally involuntary as those resulting from threats, they simultaneously tend to completely reject confessions following threats, but not those following promises. This skewed pattern of results is referred to as the positive coercion bias (Kassin, 1997).

While the Reid nine steps of interrogation protocol is possibly the best-known interrogation technique that includes some (dubious) pressure on the suspect, it is of course not the only in its sort. In the Netherlands, for example, a few decades ago, there was quite some tumult about a similar interrogation technique called communication analysing system Europe (CASE 36). In this protocol, the interrogators are assisted via ear plugs by observing colleagues in an adjacent room, watching the interrogation and observing the suspect. The suspect is shown crime scene photographs, and these are intertwined with private pictures of the suspect and his family. The suspect is told that confessing will result in a lower sentence. He is also told that his family is threatened by third parties, and that the police can only offer protection once he has confessed. At some point, the Dutch Supreme Court decided that CASE 36 is in conflict with constitutional law, and confessions obtained with this protocol should therefore not be considered as evidence.

In the current case, no registrations of the interrogations were made. It is also unknown which interrogation protocol the police had in mind. Nonetheless, the confessing female suspects have made remarks in hindsight that illustrate that some interventions may have been dubious. For example, Jane has testified that she felt pressured by the police, that she did not receive any caution before her interrogation, and that the interrogators repeatedly suggested information to her. The suspects were also told that they were allowed to go home once they confessed. Further, suspects were told that their peers had already confessed and had incriminated them in these confessions. In any case, suspects were interrogated often (up to 17 times between April 11 and May 9, 1994) and for hours on end.

11.2 False Confession Experiments

Worldwide, a number of cases have occurred in which the suspect falsely confessed to having committed a crime. In the USA, the innocence project has revealed several miscarriages of justice in which false confessions were given (see also Saks & Koehler, 2005). In Great Britain, there is the Guilford four, and the Birmingham six (Gudjonsson, 2003), and in the Netherlands, the Schiedam park murder case and the Putten murder case are infamous examples.

Obviously, it is of great importance to gain insight into the prevalence of false confessions. Gudjonsson et al. (2009) asked 24,627 high school students stemming from seven European countries, whether they had ever been interrogated by the police. Of these, 2726 confirmed this question, and of these suspects, 375 (i.e., 13.8%) claimed to have made a false confession to the police. That is a disturbingly high number. It must be appreciated that experimental research in this domain is difficult because the self-harm included in a false confession is difficult to induce ethically. Nonetheless, as discussed previously, the alt key experiment by Kassin and Kiechel (1996) was a first attempt at an experimental design with the pretence of modelling an interrogation. Of their 79 undergraduate participants, 69% signed a confession, 28% showed signs of having internalised the allegation, and 9% confabulated details about their wrongdoing. In their review of 16 experiments in this tradition, Rassin and Israëls (2014) found that of the 340 guilty participants in the experiments, 252 confessed (i.e., 74%), and of the 1559 innocent participants, no less than 707 falsely confessed (i.e., 45%).

Inbau et al. (2001) are familiar with experiments on false confessions. In reference to the alt key study (Kassin & Kiechel, 1996), they argue: ‘However, it is a tremendous leap in logic to go from persuading someone that he accidentally pushed a computer key when he did not to persuading a criminal suspect that he intentionally killed his neighbor or sexually molested his child when he did not’ (p. 426).

Also: 'Even the naïve observer should recognize the inherent motivational differences between a laboratory subject who is unable to recall which words from a list were crossed off and an actual criminal suspect who may be facing life in prison if he acknowledges committing a crime … Perhaps because of ethical considerations, many laboratory studies approach the issue of criminal interrogation in such a removed sense that the phenomenon being studied is so remotely related to the actual event that regardless of the statistical significance reported, one is left with the question, What does this prove?' (p. 444). While they have a point, it is likewise true that the social pressure applied to participants is not comparable to what the police does to suspects.

Given that ethical restrictions limit scientific possibilities, and that the experimental paradigms with which (false) confession evidence is studied are hard on the participants and the experimenters, some researchers have adopted a paradigm with which false admissions can be studied, without the strict interrogation context. Merckelbach et al. (2011) had 78 undergraduates complete the Symptoms Checklist 90 (SCL 90). Participants then completed a 5–7 min filler task (Sudokus). The experimenter then interviewed the participants about 10 of their answers on the SCL 90. However, secretly, the experimenter had changed two answers, in that a higher score was induced than given by the participant. When discussing these false answers, only 37% of the participants noticed that their answers had been twisted. This nondetecting of mismatches has been dubbed choice blindness. Sauerland et al. (2013) applied this technique to a questionnaire pertaining to criminal behaviours, ranging from torturing animals to stealing a bicycle. Sixty-seven undergraduates completed this questionnaire and were interviewed about some of their answers, 10 min later. Two of their answers had been changed, and when participants were questioned about these topics (e.g., 'Why did you do that, can you elaborate on that?'), three participants (i.e., 4.5%) did not detect either change. In their second study, 37 participants were included, and the delay between completing the questionnaire and the interview was increased to 1 week. In this instance, seven participants (i.e., 18.9%) failed to detect the alterations. In addition, 1 month later, 14 participants completed the questionnaire once more, and while they were fairly consistent in their answers on the nonmanipulated items, 5 participants (i.e., 35.7%) shifted their answer on the manipulated items. This suggests that the manipulation may have had a prolonged effect on memory.

Meanwhile, confession evidence tends to make a strong incriminating impression on legal decision makers. Indeed, this evidence is intuitively strong, because it appears implausible to confess to a crime one has not committed. Kassin and Neumann (1997) presented 62 undergraduates with 4 case vignettes, about a murder, rape, assault, and car theft. There were four versions of each case file. While in all versions, there was circumstantial evidence (control version), one version included a confession, given under some pressure and other suboptimal circumstances. In another version, the main piece of evidence was an eyewitness identification, in which the witness saw the perpetrator from some distance and with little illumination. In the third version, an indirect witness gave a personality description of the suspect as an aggressive individual with a propensity for violence. Averaged over the four different crimes, 11% of the participants convicted the suspect, given only circumstantial evidence. The percentage of convicting participants was 21% in case of the dark personality description, while conviction rates were 37% given eyewitness evidence, and 56% given a confession.

Kassin and Sukel (1997) sought to explore what happens if a confession is known to the decision maker, but inadmissible at the same time. In their first study, they presented a case vignette about a suspect called Wilson who was suspected of having killed his wife and a neighbour, to 85 undergraduates. Wilson testified that he came home, and found his wife and the neighbour dead in his house, after which he dialled the alarm number. Curiously though, he seems to have fled from the crime scene and had phoned his attorney before calling the alarm central. In four additional versions, Wilson confessed the double manslaughter after interrogation. In two of these versions, there was high social pressure during the interrogation; in the other two, pressure was low. Also, in two versions, the confession was admissible, but in the other two, it was deemed inadmissible. Participants were asked to what extent the confession had influenced their verdict, and, of course, they were asked whether they would convict Wilson. Their second study was a replication with 80 undergraduates, in which there was slightly more evidence in all five conditions (i.e., a witness saw Wilson flee the crime scene with something in his hand that looked like a knife), in order to increase conviction. Findings in both studies are summarised in Table 11.1.

As can be seen in the conviction rates, confession evidence did affect the verdict, even though participants believed that it did not. The authors conclude that it is virtually impossible to mentally exclude evidence from the decision-making process. They speculated that this unintentional influence may take place via assimilation, that is, knowledge of the confession might have inflated the perceived strength of the other incriminating evidence. If this happens, subsequent exclusion of the confession will still leave the inflated strength of the other evidence unaltered. However, they did not find evidence to suggest that participants who were knowledgeable about the confession, indeed perceived the other evidence to be stronger compared to participants in the control groups. In summary, there is reason to argue that confession evidence is intuitively strong, and can have a strong and lasting impact on conviction.

Table 11.1 Self-reported influence of confession evidence, and conviction rate as a function of admissibility (Kassin & Sukel, 1997)

		Low pressure		High pressure	
	No confession	Admissible	Inadmissible	Admissible	Inadmissible
Study 1					
Self-reported influence	–	59%	24%	41%	12%
Conviction rate	6%	29%	18%	24%	29%
Study 2					
Self-reported influence	–	68%	50%	56%	19%
Conviction rate	19%	63%	50%	50%	44%

11.3 Safeguards Against False Confessions

In many legal systems, the prevention of false confessions, and consequently false convictions is a priority. Kassin (1997) argues that 'in the context of a legal system founded on the ideal that it is better to acquit 10 guilty people than to convict 1 person who is innocent … the false positive error – although less frequent than the false negative – presents the more serious problem' (p. 224). In this light, various preventive measures can be taken to reduce the occurrence of (undetected) false confessions. One drastic solution would be to simply stop interrogating suspects. Indeed, there is a recent movement to not interrogate but interview suspects. In this investigative interview approach, the primary goal is not to obtain a confession, but to gather information. The suspect is not seen as an enemy of the police, but as a positive source of information. Hence, rapport building is crucial in this approach. Preliminary findings suggest that investigative interviewing yields better results than accusatory interrogating, in terms of fewer false confessions, but also in terms of an increase of information provided by the suspect (Meissner et al., 2014).

A less drastic intervention is to videotape suspect interrogations. Using a mock crime design, Kassin et al. (2014) found that if interrogators know that the interrogation is recorded, they tend to employ fewer minimisation and maximisation techniques. They also appear to be less eager to obtain a confession from the suspect, according to the suspects themselves. Kassin (1997) issued a few cautionary notes regarding video recording of interrogations. Particularly, even if an interrogation is recorded, mistakes can be made. First, Kassin discussed the point of view bias: If only the suspect is filmed, the observer does not get a good impression of the non-verbal behaviour of the interrogators. Therefore, it is crucial that the cameras film the complete interrogation room, not just from one angle. Second, when discussing the film in court, it should be prevented that only the final part in which the suspects confess is discussed. If so, the recap bias occurs: By solely looking at the taped confession, the observer misses the events that led up to the confession, whereas those events are what really matters. Finally, it should be acknowledged that even if an interrogation is filmed, parties (e.g., defence attorney and prosecutor) can still selectively use fragments to support their own case. For example, if the suspect at some point appears tired and emotionless, the defence can construe this as the result of prolonged wrecking interrogation, whereas the prosecutor may use the same fragment to illustrate that the suspect is a cold-hearted criminal. Hence, Kassin refers to this as the framing bias.

In addition to conducting less accusatory interviews, and/or recording interrogations, it may also be beneficial to have the defence attorney more often present during interrogations. Presence of the counsel may serve several goals, such as providing assistance to the suspect, and correcting the interrogator's behaviour, if in no other way, by having him know that he is watched (cf. the effect of video recording). Verhoeven and Stevens (2012) observed 168 interrogations, during some of which the suspect's lawyer was present. In all instances, the suspect was under suspicion of a capital crime (murder). The authors ran regression analyses, and concluded that the presence of a lawyer during the interrogation was associated with an increase of invocation of the right to remain silent, with a shortening of the interrogation length, and also with a decrease of intimidation by the interrogator (e.g., by walking around, or making bodily movements, enacting the perpetrator's behaviour). However, the authors argue that this fruitful result is quite fragile, because intimidation was in all a rarely used coercion tactic (compared to sympathizing, confrontation, and manipulation), and silent suspects tended to elicit intimidation. Hence, if a suspect is advised by his lawyer beforehand to remain silent, while the lawyer is not present during the interrogation, his silence may provoke harsh interrogation tactics.

Finally, in order to prevent false confessions, or at least to detect (increased risk of) false confessions, it may be fruitful to check whether the suspect suffers from interrogative vulnerabilities. Various factors may constitute vulnerability such as mental illness, intellectual disabilities, temporary abnormal mental states (e.g., due to sleep deprivation or intoxication), and personality characteristics. As to the latter, suggestibility is a first candidate to come to mind. Interrogative suggestibility can be defined as 'the extent to which, within a closed social interaction, people come to accept messages communicated during formal questioning, as the result of which their subsequent behavioural response is affected' (Gudjonsson, 2003, p. 345). A core feature of suggestibility is that the post hoc (mis)information is incorporated in the recollection of the receiver. Hence, subsequently, the pertinent recollection is overwritten and replaced by an altered version. Obviously, suggestibility is a vehicle by which testimonies can become corrupted. Admittedly, the success of suggestion also depends on the persuasiveness of the communicator, the credibility of the message, and the context, but the receiver's suggestibility is equally crucial. Unfortunately, suggestibility is difficult to measure, because it is hidden from introspection. Indeed, if one is aware that one has been persuaded to accept post hoc information, it would no longer be a false memory. To measure suggestibility without self-report, Gudjonsson (1984, 1997) developed the Gudjonsson Suggestibility Scale (GSS). In this test, the interviewee is presented with a short story. Next, he has to recall the story to the best of his ability. Then, 20 questions about the story are asked, 15 of which are leading, in that they presume information that was in fact not included in the story. From the free recall, a memory score and a confabulation score can be computed. From the 15 leading questions, a yield score is derived which represents the extent to which the interviewee is misled by leading questions. After a short break, the interviewer gives negative feedback including that the interviewee has made some mistakes in the first round of 20 questions. He is therefore urged to answer all questions once more. From this second round of 20 answers, a shift score is derived. That is, the number of times that the interviewee changes his second answer to the 15 leading questions, compared to the first round. This shift score represents the susceptibility to social pressure. Eventually, the yield (range: 0–15) and shift (0–15) scores are summed to produce the total suggestibility score (0–30). Higher scores represent stronger suggestibility.

Besides the popular GSS, Gudjonsson (1989) also invented the Gudjonsson Compliance Scale (GCS), that obviously measures compliance. This trait differs from suggestibility in that it is not a memory problem. A compliant witness seeks to behave in a way that he believes his conversational partner desires or expects him to do. Indeed, like suggestibility, compliance can be expected to play a role in the development of false details in witness and suspect testimonies. Also measurable is acquiescence: The preference to answer questions affirmatively (Winkler et al., 1982). This tendency can obviously be detrimental in the context of statement validity, and can be measured with a self-report in which multiple pairs of conflicting items are included. Respondents who repeatedly answer both items of a conflicting pair affirmatively display acquiescence.

In conclusion, insight into the personality traits mentioned above, and others, can strengthen the argument that a particular alternative scenario is to be taken seriously. Although the traits represent specific alternative explanations for the occurrence of incriminating testimonies, there is some overlap between some of them. For example, Gudjonsson (2003) reports significant correlations between the GSS, GCS, and a measure of acquiescence. Finally, caution is in place regarding the interpretation of scores on the pertinent scales referred to above. A high score reflects that the respondent is at increased risk to give false testimony, due to a pertinent personality trait. However, high scores are merely alarming. They cannot prove that an incriminating testimony is the result of suggestibility, compliance, and so on. Moreover, while high scores are alarming, low scores do absolutely not guarantee that the testimony given by the low scoring respondent is valid.

Geijsen et al. (2018) included 37 Dutch suspects and their interrogations in their study and made two discoveries. First, most suspects are indeed to be classified as vulnerable, in that 55.6% suffered a mental illness, 27.8% had an intellectual disability, and 11.1% had a temporary abnormal mental state (the authors did not take into account personality traits such as suggestibility, because measures such as the GSS do not have a clear cut-off score). Altogether, 69.4% of the suspects were vulnerable. Second, strikingly, the authors also concluded that only 14% of the interrogations were appropriate (e.g., absence of coercion, slow pace, stress reduction, and relative brevity). These findings suggest that there is yet much to gain from mapping suspects' vulnerabilities.

When the case of the Breda six was reopened, suspect vulnerabilities played an important role. For example, forensic psychologist Dr. Oudejans and psychiatrist Dr. van Balkom had initially concluded that Carien suffers from a retardation in her cognitive development. According to Geijsen et al. (2018), this is a vulnerability to be kept in mind, and interrogators should refrain from employing suggestive techniques.

In 2013, a colleague, Dr. Geraerts, did what she called in-depth interviews with the female suspects. She came to the conclusion that they were susceptible to social pressure and in some instances traumatised by the things they had gone through a suspect in this case, by then 20 years ago.

In 2014, I subjected the three female suspects to several tests, including the GSS and GCS. Findings were mixed. I found that Carien had elevated GSS and GCS scores, Jane had an elevated GCS (but not GSS) score, and Jenny scored low on the

GSS (and average on the GCS). Among other things, I wrote that the test scores were in my opinion more valuable than the in-depth interviews conducted by Geraerts.

Another legal psychologist, Dr. Horselenberg wrote a report about false confessions in general. He discussed the scientific literature on this topic. He also wrote that GSS and GCS scores may not reflect the suspects' personality 20 years earlier. He further mentioned that in some experiments on false confessions (including his own), GSS and GCS scores did not predict false confession. At that point in time, the meta-analysis by Otgaar et al. (2021), suggesting that GCS and particularly GSS do predict false confession proneness, had not yet seen the light.

In short, the three of us unknowingly did a good job in tackling each other's contribution, and sending mixed signals to the court that had reopened the case.

11.4 Negative Evidence

According to the confessions of the female suspects, grandma Mok was kidnapped in her own house, and was brought reluctantly and loudly to the restaurant by car. There, at some point, she was brutally abused: The men beat her, kicked her, and spat at her while she was on the floor. From an adjacent room, the females also heard multiple gun shots.

Strikingly, many of these details were not corroborated by any evidence. For example, while hair and blood drops were found next to the dead body, DNA analyses indicated that these were not from any of the suspects. Likewise, shoeprints were found on the victim's clothes (probably because she was kicked). However, none of the prints matched any shoes found in the suspects' homes. No saliva was found, although two men allegedly spat on the victim. Despite that fire arms were seen by the women, and shots were heard, none were found (no guns, ammunition, and no powder traces).

Finally, one of the crucial nova was that two people came forward who testified to have sat talking at a bus stop right in front of the restaurant, the whole night. They testified that they had noticed nothing irregular during the night. This is at odds with the primary scenario in which the six suspects violently dragged miss Mok out of their car and into the Chinese restaurant.

11.5 The End … or Is it?

Interestingly, in the course of the review of this case, the prosecution hired one more expert, Dr. Alkemade, who wrote a complete Bayesian analysis of the evidence. Although the content of this report was not made public, the conclusion was that the posterior odds in favour of the primary hypothesis are 532. Obviously, this is an incriminating outcome. The defence had a twofold argument against this. First, they hired three counter experts, Drs. Prakken, ten Hove, and van de Goot who all disagreed with Alkemade, and testified that he had made very speculative estimates of the likelihood ratios included in his report. Second, they argued that the prosecution had given only part of the casefile to Alkemade (many of the anomalies were left out). The defence was successful in this regard, and the court decided not to use Alkemade's analysis as evidence.

The Supreme Court rejected the appeals nonetheless and left the original convictions unaltered. Among other things, the court reasoned that the blood from the unknown person might be of an illegal chef, working at the restaurant. The suspects may have gotten rid of their shoes, which explains why the prints did not match any of their shoes. Indeed, 9 months had passed since the murder before the suspects' houses were searched. In all, the court acknowledged that the forensic technical analyses did not support the primary hypothesis, but they argued that it also did not contradict it: 'Absence of evidence is not evidence of absence'. In hindsight, the technical investigation was simply deemed suboptimal. As to the confessions, the court decided that they were admissible, because the experts had given inconclusive opinions, and thus, it was not convincingly argued that the confessions were unreliable. Any inconsistencies and improbabilities in the confessions were attributable to the relatively long retention period between the crime and the interrogations.

References

Geijsen, K., Vanbelle, S., Kop, N., & de Ruiter, C. (2018). The interrogation of vulnerable suspects in The Netherlands: An exploratory study. *Investigative Interviewing: Research and Practice, 9*, 34–51.

Gudjonsson, G. H. (1984). A new scale of interrogative suggestibility. *Personality and Individual Differences, 5*, 303–314.

Gudjonsson, G. H. (1989). Compliance in an interrogative situation: A new scale. *Personality and Individual Differences, 10*, 535–540.

Gudjonsson, G. H. (1997). *The Gudjonsson suggestibility scales*. Psychology Press.

Gudjonsson, G. H. (2003). *The psychology of interrogations and confessions: A handbook*. Wiley.

Gudjonsson, G. H., Sigurdsson, J. F., & Sigfusdottir, I. D. (2009). Interrogation and false confessions among adolescents in seven European countries: What background and psychological variables best discriminate between false confessors and non-false confessors? *Psychology, Crime & Law, 15*, 711–728.

Inbau, F. E., Reid, J. E., Buckley, J. P. & Jayne, B. C. (2001). *Criminal interrogation and confessions*. Gaithersburg: Aspen publishers.

Kassin, S. M. (1997). The psychology of confession evidence. *American Psychologist, 52*, 221–233.

Kassin, S. M. (2005). On the psychology of confessions: Does innocence put innocents at risk? *American Psychologist, 60*, 215–228.

Kassin, S. M., & Kiechel, K. L. (1996). The social psychology of false confessions: Compliance, internalization, and confabulation. *Psychological Science, 7*, 125–128.

Kassin, S. M., & Neumann, K. (1997). On the power of confession evidence: An experimental test of the fundamental difference hypothesis. *Law and Human Behavior, 21*, 469–484.

Kassin, S. M., & Sukel, H. (1997). Coerced confessions and the jury: An experimental test of the "harmless error" rule. *Law and Human Behavior, 21*, 27–46.

Kassin, S. M., Kukucka, J., Lawson, V. Z., & DeCarlo, J. (2014). Does video recording alter the behaviour of police during interrogation? A mock crime-and-investigation study. *Law and Human Behavior, 38*, 73–83.
Meissner, C. A., Redlich, A. D., Michael, S. W., Evans, J. R., Camiletti, C. R., Bhatt, S., & Brandon, S. (2014). Accusatorial and information-gathering interrogation methods and their effects on true and false confessions: A meta-analytic review. *Journal of Experimental Criminology, 10*, 459–486.
Merckelbach, H., Jelicic, M., & Pieters, M. (2011). Misinformation increases symptom reporting: A test-retest study. *Journal of the Royal Society of Medicine Short Reports, 2*(75), 1–6.
Otgaar, H., Schell-Leugers, J. M., Howe, M. L., De La Fuente Vilar, A., Houben, S. T. L., & Merckelbach, H. (2021). The link between suggestibility, compliance, and false confessions: A review using experimental and field studies. *Applied Cognitive Psychology, 35*, 445–455.
Rassin, E., & Israëls, H. (2014). False confessions in the lab: A review. *Erasmus Law Review, 7*, 219–224.
Saks, M. J., & Koehler, J. J. (2005). The coming paradigm shift in forensic identification science. *Science, 309*, 892–895.
Sauerland, M., Schell, J. M., Collaris, J., Reimer, N. K., Schneider, M., & Merckelbach, H. (2013). "Yes, I have sometimes stolen bikes": Blindness for norm-violating behaviors and implications for suspect interrogations. *Behavioral Sciences & the Law, 31*, 239–255.
Verhoeven, W. J., & Stevens, L. (2012). The lawyer in the Dutch interrogation room: Influence on police and suspect. *Journal of Investigative Psychology and Offender Profiling, 9*, 69–92.
Winkler, J. D., Kanouse, D. E., & Ware, J. E. (1982). Controlling for acquiescence response set in scale development. *Journal of Applied Psychology, 67*, 555–561.

Chapter 12
Mister Big and a Disputed Confession

Saturday evening December 18, 2010, Wim and Heidy are at a party. Heidy's father babysits their toddler. As the evening advances, Wim goes home to relieve his father-in-law, while Heidy stays at the party. Around midnight, a crime takes place. Wim's account is by and large as follows. At some point before midnight, he texts Heidy that all is well at home, and that he will go to bed. Heidy replies that she will soon come home. Wim falls asleep rapidly but wakes up about 30 min later, because he hears strange noises below, in the living room. He goes downstairs to check it out and finds that the room was searched. The doors to the backyard are open. He walks into the garden and sees Heidy lying on the ground, around a corner. He tries to help her, but she does not react in any way. He then calls the alarm number. Heidy has a headwound but seems to have died from strangulation.

The initial hypothesis is that their house was burgled and Heidy came home, via the garage and backyard, and was then killed by the burglar. Alternatively, the burglar may have lured in the bushes, and forced Heidy to let him into the property. And then he killed her. However, after a few days of investigation, the police come to doubt this hypothesis, for various reasons. For example, the investigators find the crime scene atypical. Cabinet drawers were open or closed in a way that was atypical for a burglary, at least according to a police crime staging expert. Apparently, nothing was stolen. Wim's housekey was found beneath Heidy's body, which remained unexplained. No technical evidence was found to suggest that an unknown person had been on the premises. Notably, it snowed the whole evening. Therefore, one would expect traces of a fight, or at least footprints, in the snow in the backyard. That said, the police did find various footprints but curiously failed to secure them (de Coninck, 2021). Further, Wim turned out to have an extramarital affair with another women. She had given him an ultimatum to choose between her and Heidy, before New Year's Eve. All this made Wim the primary suspect, after all. The police believed that he wanted to get rid of Heidy, to be with his new friend. Therefore, he killed her and then staged the burglary.

ECLI:NL:GHDHA:2022:205

E. Rassin, *Case Studies in Legal Psychology*,
https://doi.org/10.1007/978-3-031-44931-4_12

Wim denied fiercely, and stuck to his original story throughout the many interrogations he was subjected to. Although the police are strongly convinced that Wim is the murderer, they have to close the case in June 2011, and label it as unsolved. For Dutch standards, that is difficult to accept because most capital crimes are solved. Meanwhile, Wim goes on with his life. He marries his new friend, and they get a new baby. He does have problems with finding a job because employers are reluctant to take on people with dubious experiences. Two years later, things start looking sunnier when Wim gets acquainted with someone who can use a person with Wim's IT skills. This new friend is a troubleshooter who works freelance for various people. Admittedly though, some of the jobs he, and Wim do, are (semi-) illegit. For example, Wim gets paid 500 euro for a 15-minute job making a dubious film clip that is incriminating for an unspecified VIP disappear from the internet.

Things started looking really bright in 2014 when Wim and his friend were considered as candidates to do a very lucrative IT job. If they were chosen, they would earn 75,000 euro each. The person who has to decide is very rich, but earned his fortune in a dubious manner. Wim and his friend will meet him in his luxurious villa in Marbella (Spain). Wim's friend has worked for this man before, and describes him as fair but harsh. It has come to his attention that Wim has attracted police attention, and that is considered to be a liability. His friend confesses to Wim that years ago he caused a car accident while under the influence of alcohol. In that accident, his wife died. The man they are about to visit managed to steer away all police attention. No one ever found out that Wim's friend had been under the influence of alcohol. The man can do the same for Wim, but he will only initiate all this if he is convinced that it is necessary. Therefore, Wim has to come clean about his role in the death of Heidy. But Wim will not confess to this unknown rich man, because he is innocent, that is, so he says. During their audience in the villa, the man asks Wim about the death of Heidy. When Wim says to be innocent of her death, the man tells him and his friend to get out, with loud voice and swearing. In the taxi ride back to the hotel, Wim's friend makes the situation clear once more: If Wim confesses, no one will think less of him, the big boss they just met will take care of any loose ends, and the deal is on. But if Wim keeps on denying, the deal is off. At that point, Wim says that he did kill Heidy. He wanted to go live with his new love, but could not handle a divorce. Therefore, he thought it would be easier to kill Heidy. Wim's friend reassures him that when he tells this to the big boss, things will work out fine, and the deal will be on.

Days later, Wim is arrested. It turns out that the big boss is in fact an undercover police officer. So is Wim's friend. Everything that Wim experienced in the last year with his new friend was in fact an elaborated undercover operation, aimed at getting Wim to confess to Heidy's murder. Upon Wim's arrest, he immediately retracts his confession and claims that he falsely confessed merely because of the alleged gain. The operation applied in this case is known as a mister Big operation (Smith et al., 2009). Despite Wim's retraction of his confession, he is sentenced, largely because of the confession, to 18 years of imprisonment. In appeal, he even gets 20 years. A police journal devotes some attention to the case, and the undercover team is quoted cheering 'we did it, we 've got him'. But then the Supreme Court decided in 2019 that the mister Big operation was disproportionate, particularly because the undercover agent not only offered business proposals to the suspect, but also actually befriended him. Further, the court found it inappropriate that the undercover agents continued their act for days, after Wim had confessed in the taxicab. The Supreme Court decided that the whole procedure needed to be redone.

12.1 The Psychology of Confession

The court asked me for an opinion on the strength of the confession. As in the case discussed in Chap. 11, I took two concurrent approaches. First, I subjected the suspect to a handful of tests, including the GSS and the GCS. However, besides suggestibility and compliance, another personality trait might be relevant in this case. That is, under the alternative hypothesis, Wim confessed because he wanted to close the deal. Hence, he lied about his involvement in Heidy's death. Whereas the GSS and GCS are considered to be standardized tests to measure vulnerabilities, no such instrument exists to measure deceit proneness. It seems inappropriate to be critical about someone's testimony merely because that person scores high on a specific personality test. Note however that in the context of forensic mental health assessment, we do assume that people high on psychopathy are prone to deception, and other unethical behaviour. I asked the suspect to complete the Short Dark Triad (SD3; Jones & Paulhus, 2014), a measure of psychopathy, Machiavellianism, and Narcissism, traits that have been associated with deceitfulness. Wim scored low on the GSS, high on the GCS, and average to low on the SD3. Thus, Wim seemed to have one vulnerability, namely compliance.

In addition to the test strategy, I wrote in my report about the experimental literature on confession evidence. The previously mentioned alt key study (Kassin & Kiechel, 1996) and its conceptual replications were mentioned. Particularly, a study by Russano et al. (2005) was addressed. These authors sought to replicate the alt key study, while including some improvements. In their study, they had participants commit a more serious offense, namely to cheat in a test situation. This is obviously more serious than pressing the alt key in an experiment. The act of cheating can also be expected to be more intentional compared to accidentally pressing the alt key. Finally, whereas in the alt key study, all participants were in fact innocent, in the Russano et al. set-up, some were innocent and others were guilty. This allows for the estimation of diagnostic values of confessions.

Russano et al. (2005) had 296 undergraduates work on various pen-and-paper tasks in duos. Some of the problems were to be solved together, whereas others had to be solved individually. For the latter kind of problems, working together was strictly forbidden. At some point, the other participant, who was in fact a confederate, asked the participants for help with a problem that should be solved individually. Some participants let themselves be lured into working together (the guilty participants), whereas others would not cooperate (innocent suspects). When the experimenter came back into the test room, collected the answer forms, and briefly

Table 12.1 Confession likelihoods in Russano et al. (2005)

	True confession	False confession	Likelihood ratio
Standard interrogation	46%	6%	7.67
Deal	72%	14%	5.14
Minimisation	81%	18%	4.50
Deal + minimisation	87%	43%	2.02

inspected them, he would notice that both participants had the same wrong solution for an individual problem. He accused the participants of cheating, and took them apart for a brief interrogation. In this experiment, there were four interrogation protocols, inspired by the nine-step technique. In the standard condition, the suspicion of cheating was simply repeated four times. In the deal condition, participants were promised some procedural leniency ('Things could probably be settled pretty quickly'). In the minimisation condition, moral severity of the crime was reduced ('I'm sure you didn't realize what a big deal it was'). Finally, there was a condition in which the deal and the minimisation were combined. Confession rates, as a function of interrogation protocol, are presented in Table 12.1. As can be seen, findings suggest that the tricks increased, almost doubled, the likelihood of true confessions. At the same time, the likelihood of false confessions inflated even more. Consequently, the diagnostic value of the confession decreased with inclusion of the tricks. In other words, it is quite paradoxical that by inclusion of trickery, more guilty suspects are brought to confess, while simultaneously, the evidentiary power of the confession is reduced. Given that in the current case, the suspect was placed in a situation in which confessing would result in a lucrative deal, and his friend promised that he would never think less of him, I argued that the strength of the confession was weak. Moreso considering the suspect's elevated score on compliance.

12.2 The Anatomy of Criminal Conviction

How did the court come to the conviction that the suspect was guilty in the initial round? In fact, the court neatly summarises the evidence that resulted in the conviction, when 'seen in combination'. It should be kept in mind that the court not only needs to decide whether the suspect is the perpetrator, but also whether a crime occurred at all. The following pieces of evidence are listed in the verdict.

1: The report of the police officers who first came to the crime scene after Wim had called the alarm number.

2–5: Testimonies of neighbours who heard noises in the pertinent night, including a scream.

6–7: The reports of the medical examinator pertaining to Heidy's cause of death.

8: The report about forensic evidence on Heidy's clothes.

9–10: The forensic reports about (absence of) signs of burglary in the garden and on doors and windows.
11–12: Testimonies by the two undercover agents about the confession.

The court concludes that all this information points in the direction of the suspect. As such, the court accumulated all incriminating information in a one-dimensional way. In other words, they answered the question as to what extent the evidence is in line with the suspect being the perpetrator. The court made some additional typical remarks. As to the confession being elicited in an unfair manner, the court argued that in an undercover situation, the police cannot identify themselves as such, and hence cannot place pressure on the suspect in the way they can in a custodial interrogation. Therefore, the suspect need not and cannot be cautioned. And therefore, the court could not appreciate how the suspect would have come to confess due to any pressure. The defence had brought a Bayesian analysis by the hand of Derksen to the court's attention. Derksen came to a posterior odds of 0.017, with a corresponding probability of 1.7% that the suspect killed his wife. The court did not share this conclusion, and noted that the Bayesian approach to criminal evidence is disputable. Finally, the court did not see the need to investigate any alternative hypotheses, because that is only necessary if the suspect provides such an alternative. Given that Wim had confessed, any analysis of alternatives was uncalled for.

The court to which the Supreme Court had sent the case for redoing analysed the evidence in a different manner. This court chose a hypotheses-driven approach. It can even be said that their approach was Bayesian. The court starts with the remark that in order to prove that the suspect is guilty, they will have to decide between two competing hypotheses: The guilt hypothesis versus the burglar hypothesis. They also state that beforehand, the guilt hypothesis seems to be more likely. This can be construed as a qualitative prior odds. As a first constellation of evidence, the court uses the many inconsistencies in the suspect's statements (about his key found under Heidy's body, the limited time that elapsed between feeding the baby and falling in a deep sleep, and him being silent about his affair) and other anomalies (e.g., nothing was stolen, expected footprints were absent). Of all this, the court argues that it fits better under the guilt than under the burglar hypothesis. As to the forensic evidence, an expert had reported that this had a likelihood ratio of 200 in favour of the guilt hypothesis. However, this estimate leaned on various assumptions. If these assumptions were to be abandoned, the forensic evidence did not differentiate between the competing hypotheses. Further, new analyses revealed that DNA of an unknown person was found near a window at the backside of the house, near an exit from the garden where Heidy was found, and under one of her fingernails. Finally, intelligence indicated that two alternative suspects were said to have committed a burglary and to have killed the woman who had caught them in the act. By and large, this alternative account had not been investigated thoroughly. In all, the court argues that the evidence as a whole does not convincingly prove that the suspect was guilty, because there were also some indications that the burglar hypothesis was true. Eventually, Wim was acquitted. The verdict even added that this is likely to be frustrating and disappointing for relatives of the victim.

References

De Coninck, D. (2021). *Mister Big: Over een moord, onorthodoxe politiemethodes en een bekentenis*. Kritak/Lannoo.

Jones, D. N., & Paulhus, D. L. (2014). Introducing the Short Dark Triad (SD3): A brief measure of dark personality traits. *Assessment, 21*, 28–41.

Kassin, S. M., & Kiechel, K. L. (1996). The social psychology of false confessions: Compliance, internalization, and confabulation. *Psychological Science, 7*, 125–128.

Russano, M. B., Meissner, C. A., Narchet, F. M., & Kassin, S. M. (2005). Investigating true and false confessions within a novel experimental paradigm. *Psychological Science, 16*, 481–486.

Smith, S. M., Stinson, V., & Patry, M. W. (2009). Using the "Mr. Big" technique to elicit confessions: Successful innovation or dangerous development in the Canadian legal system? *Psychology, Public Policy, and Law, 15*, 168–193.

Chapter 13
Conclusion

In this book, I have discussed 11 cases in which I served as a legal psychological expert witness. Across the cases, I tried to make two points: The first is that there is scientific knowledge relevant to the evaluation of criminal evidence. That knowledge pertains to perception and memory, social influences on retrieval of recollections, the way in which interviews should and should not be conducted in order to facilitate optimal retrieval, and the dos and don'ts of identification procedures. The second point pertains to the format in which expert psychologists should ideally deliver their opinion to the court. In this conclusion, I will make a few final remarks about my analyses.

13.1 Case Studies as Starting Point of Analyses

Case studies can make a strong impression. Indeed, they reflect real events. However, case studies are scientifically limited, because they cannot prove universal laws. To that end, cleverly designed experiments are needed. Hence, the case studies in this book do not justify the conclusion that judges generally fail to appreciate the logic of eyewitness identification procedures, or the risk of false confessions. The cases were merely selected as a starting point for a discussion of the literature. It should further be noted that there probably is a selection bias in the presented cases. It seems likely that judges and lawyers will only then ask for legal psychological advice if they have doubts about the evidence. Hence, the cases in which legal psychologists are involved are not representative of typical criminal cases. There is even reason to believe that in most instances, criminal verdicts are quite valid. It is only in a minority of cases that an accumulation of flaws in the evidence and in its evaluation results in a miscarriage of justice (see Saks & Koehler, 2005).

The 11 cases discussed in this book were selected based on their suitability to introduce specific topics of legal psychological approaches to criminal evidence.

E. Rassin, *Case Studies in Legal Psychology*,
https://doi.org/10.1007/978-3-031-44931-4_13

They were selected from a pool of dozens in which I served as an expert. I found the cases by scanning a search engine (www.rechtspraak.nl) with my name as keyword. This approach reflects on two peculiarities. First, whereas suspects' names are as a general rule not mentioned in published verdicts (because of obvious privacy considerations), those of judges and experts are as a rule. Second, I was able to find many cases in which I was involved and thus found out that judges sometimes followed my advice, and sometimes did not. Hence, I found partial feedback. However, there is currently no standard procedure by which experts receive feedback from commissioning parties. Arguably, this lack of feedback hinders the expert as a learning actor.

13.2 Legal Psychology as a Forensic Expertise

Psychological science can inform legal decision makers. Sometimes laboratory findings are well in line with our intuition, for example, in case of illumination being positively related to recognition accuracy, and distance negatively (de Jong et al., 2005). In other instances, research findings contradict our previously held beliefs, for example when it comes to the exonerating power of nonidentifications (Rassin, 2013). In such cases, it may be difficult to accept the scientific insights. It may then be tempting to disqualify the scientific insights, or to reduce them to an opinion of a scientist (Bloom & Weisberg, 2007). Psychology with behaviour as its immaterial topic is more susceptible to such disqualification than for example physics (Manning et al., 2007). As mentioned earlier, it is relatively new that people have become accustomed to the idea that findings in psychological research can by deduction be used to make estimates in individual cases at all (Walker & Monahan, 1987). Against this background, I must admit that I still regularly face disbelief in my communication with lawyers and other psychological lays.

While psychological content is sometimes hard to accept, this is even worse for the hypotheses-based format that I advocate in this book. I appreciate that it is difficult to grasp that the answer to the question of whether a statement is reliable, can be that it is not, merely because it may well come forth under an alternative hypothesis. Nonetheless, there are advantages to the hypotheses approach, *in extremo*, the likelihood ratio approach. For one thing, it helps differentiate between the role of the expert (E | H), and the judge (H | E). Also, it helps to see the merits of a piece of evidence in itself, and it thus prevents premature circular arguments of the type 'the statement is reliable because it is in line with the other evidence' (cf. contextual bias). That said, legal psychologists regularly limit themselves to one-dimensional instruments like CBCA and one-dimensional opinion, and we still have a long way to go (Rassin et al., 2022). As Wagenaar (1988) wrote: 'The strategy of providing likelihoods may not solve all problems of expert testimony … the courts may interpret testimony given in the proper form as opinions thus abdicating their own responsibility of translating likelihoods into odds. A worse problem is that the experts themselves are not always fully aware of the distinction' (p. 509).

Table 13.1 Overview of possible legal psychological approaches

	Alternative hypothesis I: Deceit	Alternative hypothesis II: Mistake
Verbal/content	1	5
Nonverbal behaviour of the sender	2	6
Person(ality) of the sender	3	7
Antecedents	4	8

In summary of the various cases I was involved in, I think that my work as a legal psychologist can be categorised in a 4 * 2 table as presented in Table 13.1.

As is evident from this table, one has to consider carefully what the central argument of the alternative hypothesis is. One main category of alternatives concern deceit on the part of the source of the pertinent piece of evidence (witness or suspect). The other revolves around mistaken witness or suspect. This difference is crucial, because whereas in both cases the sender communicates incorrect information, deception requires and causes different cognitive operations than does making mistakes. For example, when lying we have to be on guard, whereas when making a mistake, we are less so because we believe to be telling the truth. This difference makes different approaches possible, even though in all instances the end result is similar, namely that the information is incorrect, and thus unsuitable to be used as evidence. For example, to start with Cell 1, a prominent way to detect deceit is the CBCA, 'probably the most widely used veracity assessment technique in the world' (Oberlader et al., 2016, p. 441). While CBCA allows for a diagnostic accuracy of approximately 70% when distinguishing truths from lies (Oberlader et al., 2016), the instrument is useless when we try to differentiate between truths and mistakes. In the words of Volbert and Steller: 'CBCA characteristics … would seem to be less appropriate for distinguishing between truthful reports and accounts based on false memories (2014, p. 215), and: "If the fabrication hypothesis is falsified because of high content quality, this does not necessarily confirm the veracity of the testimony. As pointed out above, it is also necessary to test whether it could be based on a false memory' (p. 214), and finally: 'To examine the hypothesis that a statement is based on a false memory, it is necessary to focus on the way in which the statement has emerged and evolved' (p. 207). Hence, while the use of CBCA might be considered in Cell 1 (i.e., when the alternative hypothesis is that the sender is lying), it is inappropriate in Cell 5 (i.e., when the alternative hypothesis is that the sender is mistaken). In the words of Volbert and Steller (2014, p. 208): 'a non-critical application of CBCA may well lead to a false result in these cases'.

Other verbal deception detection techniques, besides CBCA, with similar accuracy rates are the reality monitoring approach (RM; Masip et al., 2005), or simply looking for (verifiable; Nahari et al., 2014) details (Verschuere et al., 2023). While the overall accuracy of approximately 70% for verbal deception detection techniques may not be overwhelmingly impressive, these techniques may be the best option for deception detection after all. For example, the literature is quite clear that analysing nonverbal behaviour results in accuracy rates that barely differ from chance level (Bond & DePaulo, 2006, 2008). Strictly speaking, the polygraph also qualifies as a nonverbal deception detection technique, because it revolves around physiological reactions of the observed sender. These physiological reactions are small, hidden from the naked eye, but they can be detected with sensitive measurements. Crucially, while the suspect/witness is attached to the polygraph, the interviewer has various interview protocols at his disposal. Best known and most prevalent is the control/comparison question technique (CQT). The idea behind this protocol is that the suspect or witness will have to lie when answering certain self-incriminating questions (e.g., 'Did you break into this apartment?'). A guilty suspect may indeed want to falsely deny, and telling this lie will activate a defensive autonomic nervous reaction manifested in increased heart rate, blood pressure, skin conduction, breathing, pupil dilation, and even an altered P300 (EEG). Pavlidis et al. (2002) advocated that facial temperature can also be employed as physiological measure, making it possible to conduct lie detection test without personal physical contact (i.e., by remote camera), for example at airports where passengers are asked whether they have forbidden items in their luggage. Generally, these physiological changes associated with lying will show in the polygraph output. After approximately 25 s, the physiological processes will have returned to baseline level (the P300 is normalised after no more than 2 s; Ben-Shakhar, et al., 2002). Theoretically, lies will show in the output, whereas truthful answers do not result in altered physiological reactions. This way, liars will be differentiated from truth-tellers. It must be acknowledged, however, that truth-tellers may also produce a guilty pattern of physiological reactions. It is feasible that an innocent suspect will be startled by the question 'Did you break into the apartment?', and will therefore react physiologically. To control for these kinds of false-positive guilty reactions, the interview protocol includes control questions (hence, the name CQT) that are emotionally arousing and elicit false answers. A possible control question in a breaking-and-entry case would be 'Have you ever stolen anything, prior to becoming a suspect in this case?'. Arguably, innocent suspects will be tempted to lie, and answer that they never have (assumption then is that all people steel something during their lives), because admitting to have stolen in the past may make a dishonest impression. Consequently, innocent suspects may show a physiological response to relevant questions, but also to control questions. Thus, their overall response pattern is relatively flat. By contrast, the response pattern of liars is characterised by peaks (in reaction to relevant questions) and (relative) valleys (in reaction to control questions). It should be noted that the CQT leans on some dubious assumptions, such as that innocents will lie to control questions (Lilienfeld & Landfield, 2008). Further, the specificity of the protocol largely depends on the strength of the control questions. The exact psychometric properties of the CQT are difficult to determine, but its sensitivity is estimated at approximately 85%, while its specificity is somewhat disappointing with 60% (e.g., Gannon et al., 2008; Patrick & Iacono, 1989).

While legal systems that allow polygraph testing as criminal evidence mostly employ the CQT, academic psychologists have become increasingly interested in an alternative interview protocol, called the guilty knowledge test (GKT), or concealed information test (CIT), also referred to as memory detection. The theory behind this protocol is slightly different from the CQT. Here, it is assumed that the actual suspect/witness will have specific detailed knowledge about the crime under investigation, because he was at the crime scene. An innocent suspect does not have this crime-specific information. In the GKT, the suspect is confronted with multiple choice questions, and with the alternative answer options (e.g., 'Did the perpetrator loose at the crime scene: 1) his weapon, 2) a shoe, 3) a key, 4) a handkerchief, 5) coins, or 6) a pen?'). It is assumed that only the guilty suspect knows the correct answer, and will therefore display an elevated physiological reaction after hearing the correct answer. This reaction is an orienting response, which is similar to the defensive response relied on in the CQT, except for the heart rate that may decrease rather than increase (see Verschuere et al., 2004). The responses are continually registered, and hence, it is evident from the polygraph output if the suspect displays a peak reaction after being confronted with the correct answer. Note that statistically, displaying a physiological peak coincidentally while not knowing the correct answer, right at the moment that the correct answer is read aloud, is only one-in-six, if six serious answer options are included after the question (i.e., 17%). Consequently, the probability of displaying a guilty peak reaction in two subsequent questions, while not having guilty knowledge, is only (17% * 17% =) 3%. Given this interview protocol, the GKT can be expected to be quite selective: When innocent, the likelihood of being falsely accused of possessing crime relevant information is small. This theoretical advantage over the CQT is also borne out from validation studies. In a meta-analysis of GKT studies, MacLaren (2001) concluded that the GKT has 76% sensitivity and 83% specificity. In their meta-analysis, Ben-Shakhar and Elaad (2003) produced medium to large effect sizes ($1.55 < d < 3.12$).

In conclusion, while the CQT is more popular in practice than is the GKT, the reverse is true for their popularity among scientists. The GKT has a better theoretical foundation, is less confronting because it seeks relevant knowledge rather than lies, does actually not even require that the suspect answers the questions (he merely needs to listen to the answers), and crucially has better psychometric properties (the likelihood ratio of a positive CQT outcome is arguably (85%: 40% =) 2.1, while that of the GKT is (76%: 17% =) 4.5). The diagnostic qualities of both protocols might be considered disappointing, particularly considering that polygraph testing requires quite some preparation and expensive equipment. A free side effect of both protocols is the bogus pipeline effect: The mere prospect of being subjected to a polygraph test makes some individuals come clean and confess in advance (Gannon et al., 2008).

The third approach is to take into account the person(ality) of the sender. In (Dutch) jurisprudence, reference to the sender's person is made occasionally. For example, when it comes to the credibility of an alibi provided by a witness, this alibi is taken seriously more readily if it is provided by a witness unrelated to the suspect, compared to when it is provided by a close friend of the suspect. In such a case, the credibility is simply made conditional upon the person of the sender. It would be of interest to know whether certain personality traits can predict whether someone would lie in case of potential gain. These traits could then be used in the context of credibility assessment. While it may seem incorrect to judge a statement to be unreliable, merely because it was given by a person scoring high on a specific test, this is principally what psychologists do in all sorts of contexts. Educational differentiation is based on test scores. Job assessment procedures involve test scores. Forensic mental health diagnostics are based on test scores. In all these cases, attempts are made to predict (future) behaviour with psychological tests. In a recent study, Rassin et al. (2023) placed undergraduates in a context in which they could cheat in a game, thinking that their cheating would go undetected, and would increase their likelihood of winning extra monetary reward. Participants had also completed a test of psychopathy, the Triarchic Psychopathy Measure (TriPM; van Dongen et al., 2017). Thirty-one (i.e., 19%) of the 166 participants cheated, that is, they exaggerated their performance by claiming that they had solved puzzles that were in fact unsolvable. These cheating participants scored higher on the TriPM than did the 135 honest participants. The distributions of TriPM scores are displayed in Fig. 13.1.

It is easy to see how this information might assist in credibility assessment. Imagine that a decision maker has the impression that a certain statement may be false (e.g., based on verbal characteristics). Imagine then that it is known that the sender scores between 70 and 79 on this measure. Potential liars have an eight times higher likelihood of reaching this score. Hence, this test score may be informative. Besides psychopathy, other dark traits such as Machiavellianism, narcissism, and sadism are potential candidates for the prediction of deception (Paulhus et al., 2021).

Finally, as to Cell number 4, little is known about the diagnosticity of antecedents for the determination of truthfulness. Obviously, one may consider whether there are obvious reasons to lie borne out by the case file (e.g., revenge). However, to the best of my knowledge, nothing is known about the diagnosticity of such endeavours.

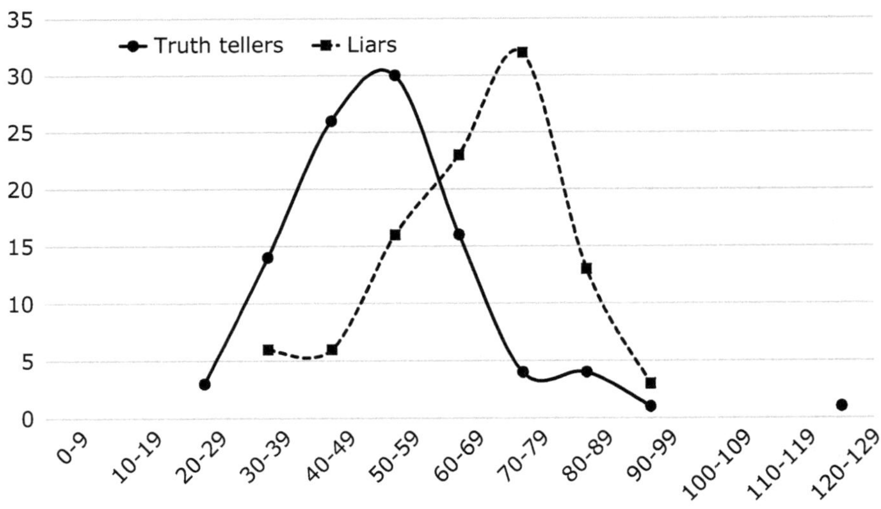

Fig. 13.1 Distribution of TriPM scores of honest and deceitful participants. (Rassin et al., 2023)

The second alternative hypothesis, in which the sender is genuine but mistaken, has its own opportunities and limitations. Whereas verbal analyses have their strengths in case of suspected deceit, they are virtually useless and inappropriate in case of suspected mistakes (Cell 5 in Table 13.1). Obviously, if there are bizarre details or details that indisputably prove that the statement is true, the content is of importance. However, if the opinion of a legal psychologist is solicited, there is probably no obvious cue in the content of the pertinent statement that helps to determine its truthfulness. In those cases, psychology does not offer tools or criteria to distinguish accurate narratives from those based on a false memory. Particularly, our lively imagination can make false memories as lively as accurate ones (Johnson et al., 1988; Suengas & Johnson, 1988). A verbal cue that has been associated with truthfulness (as opposed to being mistaken) is self-reported confidence, particularly in the context of eyewitness identification procedures (Sporer et al.; 1995; Wells et al., 2020).

The same problem, namely that we are unaware of the falsity of some of our recollections, hinders their detection when looking for nonverbal cues (Cell 6). We genuinely react equally emotionally and physiologically to false memories as to actually experienced events (McNally et al., 2004). A nonverbal cue that may help differentiate between correct and mistaken eyewitness identifications is decision speed. Correct identifications are generally made faster than incorrect ones. Dunning and Perretta (2002) even argue that a 12 seconds cutoff might be considered.

As to Cell 7, there are various personality characteristics relevant to the development of false memories. These characteristics are commonly referred to as vulnerabilities. For example, low intelligence, mental health problems, suggestibility, and compliance are considered to put people at increased risk of giving false testimony or even false confession when placed in an interrogative context (Geijsen et al., 2018; Otgaar et al., 2021). Suggestibility and to a lesser extent compliance have also been associated with memory flaws in the context of witness statements (Rassin, 2022). Hence, it is important that these personality traits are tested and documented. For example, if a witness scores high on suggestibility, and the crucial information is only elicited from this witness after leading questions, this combination gives weight to the alternative hypothesis. Many but not all potentially relevant traits are by now measurable (e.g., Gudjonsson, 1984, 1989; Winkler et al., 1982).

Finally, as opposed to the situation in which the alternative hypothesis revolves around deceit (Cell 4), an analysis of antecedents is highly relevant in case of suspected mistakes (Cell 8). In my experience, analyses of antecedents to shed light on possible sources of mistakes are the most prominent contribution of legal psychologists. In fact, when it comes to the potential of mistakes, everything from the moment of the alleged incident until the police interview in which the pertinent statement is given is of essence. To start, a correct statement (or identification) requires that the pertinent incident was perceived well in the first place. Many external circumstances, such as distance, illumination, angle, and exposure duration, effect the quality of the perception and hence of the later reproduction (e.g., de Jong et al., 2005). In addition, internal factors such as attention (Deffenbacher, 1985; Drew et al., 2013) or alcohol consumptions (van Oorsouw & Merckelbach, 2012) play a role. After sufficient perception, the recollection has to be stored for a while. Problem here is that accurate recollections tend to fade over time, making them more similar to internally generated imaginations (Johnson et al., 1988; Suengas & Johnson, 1988). Consequently, it is more difficult to distinguish accurate from false recollections based on their characteristics when they pertain to the distant past, compared to when they are recent. If for no other reason, this fading makes retention time unfortunate, credibility-wise. Longer retention times also increase the possibilities for spontaneous reconstruction (Roediger & McDermott, 1995), as well as for interaction with third parties during which post hoc information is suggested. Finally, the recollection has to be retrieved in its most authentic form, which is why suggestions are detrimental. By now, there is ample reason to argue that around one-third of participants will fall prey to suggestive questions (Rassin, 2022). The effect of suggestion does not seem to be limited to a simple affirmation of the suggested information, but can actually cause rich false memories (Arce et al., 2023) of complete events, and even repeated events (Calado et al., 2021).

In sum, it is utmost important to understand which alternative hypothesis is targeted, and which approach is taken, in order to prevent misunderstanding between the legal psychologist and the legal commissioning parties.

13.3 Hypotheses-Driven Decision Making

It is valuable to stress that the argument that (psychological) experts should adhere to a hypothesis driven or even likelihood ratio approach does not necessarily imply that courts should adopt a full Bayesian approach. Likelihood ratios do appear in a Bayesian analysis, but they can also exist on their own, outside of a Bayesian context (de Keijser & Elffers, 2012; Dienes, 2008; Fenton et al., 2016; Rassin et al., 2022; Royall, 1997). However, I do advocate that judges (and juries) adopt a scenario approach in that they do not simply accumulate evidence against the suspect, but analyse every piece of evidence as to its fit in competing scenario's, even without trying to actually quantify these fits with likelihoods. Note that while I use the terms hypothesis and scenario interchangeably, some argue that a scenario is an elaborated hypothesis. In the domain of intelligence analyses, Heuer (1999) termed this approach an Analysis of Competing Hypotheses (ACH). It has also been forwarded as a fruitful way of legal decision making (van Koppen & Mackor, 2020). The crucial advantage of hypotheses-driven decision making is that it allows for the realization that evidence may not be specific for the primary hypothesis. As such, it is a derivate of the principle of falsification as common in science (cf. Popper, 1959, 1963). There is reason to argue that fact finding in science and in law should not be as different as they are currently in practice.

The effect of this approach can be seen in the last case, of Wim (Chap. 12). In the one-dimensional approach employed in the initial procedure, Wim was convicted because ample pieces of evidence supported the guilt hypothesis. However, in the second round, the court realized that much of the evidence simultaneously fitted in the alternative hypothesis. Further, evidence that was an anomaly under the primary hypothesis, and thus discarded as irrelevant in the initial procedure, seemed to fit well in the alternative hypothesis, and was thus acknowledged to be exonerating in the second round.

Strikingly though, the scientific evidence for the effect of hypotheses-driven decision making is still limited. As discussed in Chap. 1, O'Brien (2009) gave a case description about a shooting to 108 undergraduate students. In this story, there were multiple potential suspects, but one, Bill Briggs, was incriminated most by circumstantial evidence. After reading the case, some participants were asked to register their initial impression about who the perpetrator was. Then, they could select additional lines of investigation from a list of 25, some of which were incriminating for Briggs, whereas others were aimed at findings evidence against another suspect. Findings indicated that participants who were initially under the impression that Briggs was guilty selected more ($M = 1.65$) guilt confirming investigations than did those who had not expressed their initial suspicion ($M = 1.31$; $p < 0.05$). In a second study ($N = 109$ undergraduates), part of the participants again expressed their initial suspicion, but some of them also had to list three other potential suspects. Others had to list, besides their initial suspicion, reasons why they might be mistaken and why the primary suspect could be innocent. Hence, there were four conditions. As to the number of subsequently selected investigations aimed at gathering more evidence against Briggs, participants in the control condition selected on average 1, those in the initial hypothesis condition 1.48, those who had additionally listed three alternative suspects 1.54, and those who had thought of reasons why the suspect might be innocent 1.07. These data suggest that considering alternative suspects did not suppress confirmation proneness, whereas thinking of counterarguments for one's hypothesis did. Arguably, it is understandable that decision makers will become more eager to find evidence against the primary suspect after having considered three alternative suspects. Meanwhile, considering counterarguments can be construed as a form of alternative scenario thinking. It should be noted that in some legal systems, it is made difficult if not impossible for the defence to argue that there are alternative suspects (Findley & Scott, 2006; Liebman et al., 2012–2013).

At first sight, O'Brien's (2009) findings suggest that thinking of counterarguments may offer better protection against confirmation bias than does generating three alternative hypotheses. Crucially, O'Brien employed a selective exposure paradigm as a proximation of confirmation bias, which goes back to a classic study by Snyder and Swann (1978). They asked a sample of female undergraduates to conduct a short interview with someone they had never met. Half of the interviewers were to find out whether the interviewee was an extravert, the other half were given the mission to find out whether the interviewee was introverted. Participants were given a list of 26 questions from which they could select 12 to be asked during the interview. Eleven of the questions in the pool were extraversion-confirming (e.g., 'What would you do if you wanted to liven things up at a party?'), 10 were introversion-confirming (e.g., 'What things do you dislike about loud parties?'), and 5 were neutral (e.g., 'What kinds of charities do you like to contribute to?'). As expected, participants in the extraversion hypothesis condition selected many extraversion-confirming questions (i.e., 7.43) compared to introversion-directed (2.66) and neutral questions (1.91). By contrast, those in the introversion condition primarily selected introversion-confirming questions (5.77) as opposed to extraversion (4.6) and neutral ones (1.63). Eventually, the interviews were audiotaped. Twelve undergraduates listened to the interviewees' answers to six of the questions posed during the interview. They rated the interviewees on various 6-pointscales. Strikingly, on average, the interviewees in the extraversion hypothesis condition (who had been asked many hypothesis-confirming questions) were judged to be more extraverted, confident, and energetic than were their peers in the introversion hypothesis condition. These findings suggest that confirmatory strategy selection (or positive testing; Klayman, & Ha, 1987) is actually preferred, and that it may indeed result in bias.

Given the apparent limited effect of alternative hypotheses thinking as evidenced by the results of O'Brien (2009), Rassin (2018) sought to explore whether it helps to literally type out the two competing hypotheses and to score the fit of each piece of evidence within both hypotheses. Undergraduates read one of three versions of a murder story. One third of the participants read a version in which the possible motive for the suspect was added, one third read a version in which both that motive and alternative suspects were presented, and one third read the latter version, and was subsequently instructed to rate 20 pieces of information as to their fit in the primary and in the alternative scenario, on a scale from 0 through 10. Finally, participants decided whether Eva should be convicted. In the motive condition, conviction rate was 36%. In the mixed motive and alternative suspect condition, conviction rate was suppressed to 22%, but this decrease was not statistically significant. In the pen-and-paper tool condition, conviction rate was significantly suppressed to 5% ($p < 0.001$). Thus, these findings suggest that considering an alternative does suppress conviction.

Schmittat et al. (2021) presented a crime story to a mixed sample of law students and lawyers. In one version, an alternative hypothesis was added. The effect of this addition was measured on an 8-pointscale measuring perceived guilt (0 = *not at all likely*; 7 = *very likely*), and on conviction rate, amongst others. As expected, addition of the alternative hypothesis suppressed perceived guilt from 5.71 to 3.74, and conviction rate from 49% to 17%. In a second study, these results were replicated, but here, a third condition was included in which participants received a plea by the defence stating that the suspect was innocent. This plea suppressed perception of guilt (from 6.5 to 5.68) and conviction rate (from 49% to 29%) to a similar extent as did the alternative hypothesis (perceived guilt = 5.0, conviction rate = 23%). While the authors had hypothesised that the plea would be less effective, they realised afterwards that the plea included many arguments that also hinted at an alternative hypothesis.

Finally, Maegherman et al. (2021) presented a crime story to 191 undergraduates, and subsequently asked them to select 6 possible additional investigation activities from a pool of 24, of which 12 were incriminating to the primary suspect, and 12 were directed at an alternative hypothesis and were thus exonerating. Half of the participants were, prior to the study, educated about analyses of competing hypotheses (ACH). These participants turned out to select only two incriminating endeavours, and four exonerating ones. However, participants in the control condition, who had not been informed about the importance of ACH, did exactly the same: They too selected only two incriminating and four exonerating investigative endeavours. Thus, the instruction about ACH had no effect.

In sum, so far it seems that in some studies, the alternative hypotheses approach is found to make decision makers more conservative (Rassin, 2018; Schmittat et al., 2021). In others, the effect of considering alternatives is less strong than that of bluntly conjuring up reasons for why the primary hypothesis may be incorrect (O'Brien, 2009). And some studies are inconclusive, because the participants in the control condition were not biased in the first place, which precludes any effect of hypothesis-driven thinking (Maegherman et al., 2021). As always, more research is needed.

References

Arce, R., Selaya, A., Sanmarco, J., & Fariña, F. (2023). Implanting rich autobiographical false memories: Meta-analysis for forensic practice and judicial judgment making. *International Journal of Clinical and Health Psychology, 23*. https://doi.org/10.1016/j.ijchp.2023.100386

Ben-Shakhar, G., & Elaad, E. (2003). The validity of psychophysiological detection of information with the guilty knowledge test: A meta-analytic review. *Journal of Applied Psychology, 88*, 131–151.

Ben-Shakhar, G., Bar-Hillel, M., & Kremnitzer, M. (2002). Trial by polygraph: Reconsidering the use of the guilty knowledge technique in court. *Law and Human Behavior, 26*, 527–541.

Bloom, P., & Weisberg, D. S. (2007). Childhood origins of adult resistance to science. *Science, 316*, 996–997.

Bond, C. F., & DePaulo, B. M. (2006). Accuracy of deception judgments. *Personality and Social Psychology Review, 10*, 214–234.

Bond, C. F., & DePaulo, B. M. (2008). Individual differences in judging deception: Accuracy and bias. *Psychological Bulletin, 134*, 477–492.

Calado, B., Luke, T. J., Connolly, D. A., Landstrom, S., & Otgaar, H. (2021). Implanting false autobiographical memories for repeated events. *Memory, 29*(10), 1320–1341.

De Jong, M., Wagenaar, W. A., Wolters, G., & Verstijnen, I. M. (2005). Familiar face recognition as a function of distance and illumination: A practical tool for use in the courtroom. *Psychology, Crime & Law, 11*, 87–97.

De Keijser, J., & Elffers, H. (2012). Understanding of forensic expert reports by judges, defense lawyers and forensic professionals. *Psychology, Crime and Law, 18*, 191–207.

Deffenbacher, K. A. (1985). Eyewitness recall, the Yerkes-Dodson law, and optimal-level theory. *Medicine and Law, 4*, 361–372.

Dienes, Z. (2008). *Understanding psychology as a science: An introduction to scientific and statistical inferences*. Palgrave Macmillan.

Drew, T., Võ, M. L. H., & Wolfe, J. M. (2013). The invisible gorilla strikes again: Sustained inattentional blindness in expert observers. *Psychological Science, 24*, 1848–1853.

Dunning, D., & Perretta, S. (2002). Automaticity and eyewitness accuracy: A 10-to-12-seconds rule for distinguishing accurate from inaccurate positive identifications. *Journal of Applied Psychology, 87*, 951–962.

Fenton, N., Neil, M., & Berger, D. (2016). Bayes and the law. *Annual Review of Statistics and Its Application, 3*, 51–77.

Findley, K. A., & Scott, M. S. (2006). The multiple dimensions of tunnel vision in criminal cases. *Wisconsin Law Review, 2*, 291–397.

Gannon, T. A., Beech, A. R., & Ward, T. (2008). Does the polygraph lead to better risk prediction for sexual offenders? *Aggression and Violent Behavior, 13*, 29–44.
Geijsen, K., Vanbelle, S., Kop, N., & de Ruiter, C. (2018). The interrogation of vulnerable suspects in The Netherlands: An exploratory study. *Investigative Interviewing: Research and Practice, 9*, 34–51.
Gudjonsson, G. H. (1984). A new scale of interrogative suggestibility. *Personality and Individual Differences, 5*, 303–314.
Gudjonsson, G. H. (1989). Compliance in an interrogative situation: A new scale. *Personality and Individual Differences, 10*, 535–540.
Heuer, R. J. (1999). Psychology of intelligence analyses. CIA.
Johnson, M. K., Foley, M. A., Suengas, A. G., & Raye, C. L. (1988). Phenomenal characteristics of memories for perceived and imagined autobiographical events. *Journal of Experimental Psychology: General, 117*, 371–376.
Klayman, J., & Ha, Y. W. (1987). Confirmation, disconfirmation, and information in hypothesis testing. *Psychological Review, 94*, 211–228.
Liebman, J. S., Blackburn, S., Mattern, D., & Waisnor, J. (2012–2013). The evidence of things not seen: Non-matches as evidence of innocence. *Iowa Law Review, 98*, 577–688.
Lilienfeld, S. O., & Landfield, K. (2008). Science and pseudoscience in law enforcement: A user-friendly primer. *Criminal Justice and Behavior, 35*, 1215–1230.
MacLaren, V. V. (2001). A quantitative review of the guilty knowledge test. *Journal of Applied Psychology, 86*, 674–683.
Maegherman, E., Ask, K., Horselenberg, R., & van Koppen, P. J. (2021). Test of the analysis of competing hypotheses in legal decision-making. *Applied Cognitive Psychology, 35*, 62–70.
Manning, R., Levine, M., & Collins, A. (2007). The kitty Genovese murder and the social psychology of helping. *American Psychologist, 62*, 555–562.
Masip, J. M., Sporer, S. L., Garrido, E., & Herrero, C. (2005). The detection of deception with the reality monitoring approach: A review of the empirical evidence. *Psychology, Crime & Law, 11*, 99–122.
McNally, R. J., Lasko, N. B., Clancy, S. A., Macklin, M. L., Pitman, R. K., & Orr, S. P. (2004). Psychophysiological responding during script-driven imagery in people reporting abduction by space aliens. *Psychological Science, 15*, 493–497.
Nahari, G., Vrij, A., & Fisher, R. P. (2014). The verifiability approach: Countermeasures facilitate its ability to discriminate between truths and lies. *Applied Cognitive Psychology, 28*, 122–128.
O'Brien, B. (2009). Prime suspect: An examination of factors that aggravate and counteract confirmation bias in criminal investigations. *Psychology, Public Policy, and Law, 15*, 315–334.
Oberlader, V. A., Naefgen, C., Koppehele-Gossel, J., Quinten, L., Banse, R., & Schmidt, A. F. (2016). Validity of content-based techniques to distinguish true and fabricated statements: A meta-analysis. *Law and Human Behavior, 40*, 440–457.
Otgaar, H., Schell-Leugers, J. M., Howe, M. L., De La Fuente Vilar, A., Houben, S. T. L., & Merckelbach, H. (2021). The link between suggestibility, compliance, and false confessions: A review using experimental and field studies. *Applied Cognitive Psychology, 35*, 445–455.
Patrick, C. J., & Iacono, W. G. (1989). Psychopathy, threat, and polygraph test accuracy. *Journal of Applied Psychology, 74*, 347–355.
Paulhus, D. L., Buckels, E. E., Trapnell, P. D., & Jones, D. N. (2021). Screening for dark personalities: The short dark tetrad (SD4). *European Journal of Psychological Assessment, 37*(3), 208–222.
Pavlidis, I., Eberhardt, N. L., & Levine, J. A. (2002). Seeing through the face of deception: Thermal imaging offers a promisisng hands-off approach to mass security screening. *Nature, 415*, 35.
Popper, K. (1959). *The logic of scientific discovery*. Routledge.
Popper, K. (1963). *Conjectures and refutations*. Routledge.
Rassin, E. (2013). Presence bias and the insensitivity to the diagnosticity of nonidentifications. *Psychology, Crime & Law, 19*, 203–214.
Rassin, E. (2018). Reducing tunnel vision with a pen-and-paper tool for the weighting of criminal evidence. *Journal of Investigative Psychology and Offender Profiling, 15*, 227–233.

Rassin, E. (2022). Suggested false memories of a non-existent film: Forensically relevant individual differences in the *crashing memories* paradigm. *Memory, 30*(9), 1205–1211.

Rassin, E., Arbiyah, N., Boskovic, I., Otgaar, H., & Merckelbach, H. (2022). Likelihood ratios in psychological expert opinion, and their reception by professional judges. *International Journal of Evidence and Proof, 26*(4), 325–341.

Rassin, E., Sergiou, C., Van der Linden, D., & Van Dongen, J. (2023). Psychopathy as a predisposition to lie hedonistically. *Psychology, Crime & Law.* https://doi.org/10.1080/1068316X.2023.2213802

Roediger, H. L., & McDermott, K. B. (1995). Creating false memories: Remembering words not presented in lists. *Journal of Experimental Psychology: Learning, Memory and Cognition, 24*, 803–814.

Royall, R. (1997). *Statistical evidence: A likelihood paradigm*. Chapman & Hall.

Saks, M. J., & Koehler, J. J. (2005). The coming paradigm shift in forensic identification science. *Science, 309*, 892–895.

Schmittat, S. M., Englich, B., Sautner, L., & Velten, P. (2021). Alternative stories and the decision to prosecute: An applied approach against confirmation bias in criminal prosecution. *Psychology, Crime & Law*, 1–28.

Snyder, M., & Swann, W. B. (1978). Hypothesis-testing processes in social interaction. *Journal of Personality and Social Psychology, 36*, 1202–1212.

Sporer, S. L., Penrod, S. D., Read, J. D., & Cutler, B. L. (1995). Choosing, confidence, and accuracy: A meta-analysis of the confidence-accuracy relation in eyewitness identification studies. *Psychological Bulletin, 118*, 315–327.

Suengas, A. G., & Johnson, M. K. (1988). Qualitative effects of rehearsal on memories for perceived and imagined complex events. *Journal of Experimental Psychology: General, 117*, 377–389.

Van Dongen, J. D. M., Drislane, L. E., Nijman, H., Soe-Agnie, S. E., & van Marle, H. J. C. (2017). Further evidence for reliability and validity of the Triarchic psychopathy measure in a forensic sample and a community sample. *Journal of Psychopathology and Behavioural Assessment, 39*, 58–66. https://doi.org/10.1007/s10862-016-9567-5

Van Koppen, P. J., & Mackor, A. R. (2020). A scenario-approach to the Simonshaven case. *Topics in Cognitive Science, 12*, 1132–1151.

Van Oorsouw, K., & Merckelbach, H. (2012). The effects of alcohol on crime-related memories: A field study. *Applied Cognitive Psychology, 26*(1), 82–90. https://doi.org/10.1002/acp.1799

Verschuere, B., Crombez, G., de Clercq, A., & Koster, E. H. W. (2004). Autonomic responding to concealed information: Differentiating orienting and defensive responses. *Psychophysiology, 41*, 461–466.

Verschuere, B., Lin, C. C., Huismann, S., Kleinberg, B., Willemse, M., Chong Jia Mei, E., Van Goor, T., Löwy, L. H. S., Appiah, O. K., & Meijer, E. (2023). The use-the-best heuristic facilitates deception detection. *Nature Human Behaviour*. https://doi.org/10.1038/s41562-023-01556-2

Volbert, R., & Steller, M. (2014). Is this testimony truthful, fabricated, or based in false memory? Credibility assessment 25 years after Steller and Köhnken (1989). *European Psychologist, 19*, 207–220.

Wagenaar, W. A. (1988). The proper seat: A Bayesian discussion of the position of expert witnesses. *Law and Human Behavior, 12*(4), 499–510.

Walker, L., & Monahan, J. (1987). Social frameworks: A new use of social science in law. *Virginia Law Review, 73*, 559–598.

Wells, G. L., Bull Kovera, M., Douglass, A. B., Brewer, N., Meissner, C. A., & Wixted, J. T. (2020). Policy and procedure recommendations for the collection and preservation of eyewitness identification evidence. *Law and Human Behavior, 44*, 3–36.

Winkler, J. D., Kanouse, D. E., & Ware, J. E. (1982). Controlling for acquiescence response set in scale development. *Journal of Applied Psychology, 67*, 555–561.

Index

A
Allegation of sexual abuse, 63
Analysis of competing hypotheses (ACH), 68, 150, 152, 153
Anatomically detailed drawings, 100–104

B
Bayes, 5
Bayesian approach, 5, 7, 8, 16, 19, 61, 141, 150

C
Children's memories, 93, 94
Clinical heuristics, 112
Confession evidence, 1, 20, 120, 129, 130, 139
Credibility assessment, 67, 148
Criteria-Based Content Analysis (CBCA), 19, 23, 63–68, 72, 73, 144, 145

D
Dissociation, 84, 86

E
Estimator variables, 33–34, 52, 58
Expert witness, 1, 2, 19–26, 38, 63, 75, 143
Eyewitness identification, 4, 8, 10, 12, 19, 32, 52, 58–60, 129, 143, 149

F
Fact finding, 1–3, 13, 19, 31, 75, 126, 150
False memories, 67, 69, 75–79, 90, 94, 100, 132, 145, 149, 150

I
Interrogation, 20, 115, 119, 124–133, 135, 138, 140, 141

L
Legal decision making, 3–20, 150
Likelihood ratio (LR), 5, 6, 8, 16, 22–25, 39, 47, 52, 53, 58–60, 140, 141, 144, 147, 150
Line up, 22, 32–35, 37–53, 59, 60

M
Memory enhancement, 108–109
Memory interpretation, 69
Memory loss, 109, 118, 119
Mister Big, 137–141
Mugshots, 2, 31–36, 40, 41, 60

N
Negative evidence, 10, 41, 53, 118, 134
Nonverbal deception detection, 116, 146

E. Rassin, *Case Studies in Legal Psychology*,
https://doi.org/10.1007/978-3-031-44931-4

P
Peer influence, 95
Psychodynamics, 68, 69, 84, 118
Psychotherapy, 63–79, 84, 104

R
Repression, 63–79, 84

S
Sexual abuse, 65, 66, 75, 83, 86, 97
Show up, 32, 35, 36, 38–40, 42, 51, 52
Statement validity, 65, 133
Suggestive questioning, 120
Symptom validity tests (SVT), 116–118
System variables, 33, 38, 52

T
Trauma, 69, 73–75, 83–86

U
Undercover operations, 138

MIX
Papier aus verantwortungsvollen Quellen
Paper from responsible sources
FSC® C105338

If you have any concerns about our products,
you can contact us on
ProductSafety@springernature.com

In case Publisher is established outside the EU,
the EU authorized representative is:
Springer Nature Customer Service Center GmbH
Europaplatz 3, 69115 Heidelberg, Germany

Printed by Libri Plureos GmbH
in Hamburg, Germany